Control for Epilepsy Suppression: A Mathematical Treatise

Azhar ul Haque Sario

Copyright

First Printing, 2025

Azhar.sario@hotmail.co.uk

ORCID: https://orcid.org/0009-0004-8629-830X
LinkedIn: https://www.linkedin.com/in/azharulhaquesario/

Disclaimer: This book is free from AI use. The cover was designed in Microsoft PowerPoint.

Contents

The Architecture of Chaos: Spectral Graph Theory and Structural Connectivity

The Whispering City: Decoding the Geometry of a Seizure

We often speak of epilepsy with violent metaphors. We call it a "storm," a "short-circuit," or "chaos." But this language betrays a misunderstanding of the enemy.

In my work mapping the topography of the brain, I have found that a seizing brain is not broken. On the contrary, it is a machine working with terrifying perfection. It is a hyper-efficient network doing exactly what neurons are designed to do—synchronize—but at a scale that wipes out consciousness.

To understand this, we must stop looking at the brain as a biological organ and start viewing it as an architecture.

1. The Metropolis of the Mind

Imagine your brain is a sprawling, bioluminescent megacity.

The Citizens (V): These are your neurons, clustered in neighborhoods like the Hippocampus (the archives) or the Visual Cortex (the cinema).

The Highways (E): These are the white matter tracts—thick bundles of fiber-optic cables that physically connect the neighborhoods.

In a healthy city, the noise is diverse. The business district hums with commerce, the parks are quiet, the stadium creates a roar. This variety is what we call consciousness.

Epilepsy is when the traffic lights synchronize. Suddenly, every car, in every neighborhood, turns left at the exact same second. The complex jazz of the city is replaced by a singular, deafening marching beat. And here is the crucial realization: The march can only happen where the roads exist. The seizure follows the pavement.

2. The Laplacian: The Traffic Control Algorithm

To predict where the march will go, we leave metaphors and enter the realm of Spectral Graph Theory. Our primary tool is the Laplacian Matrix (L).

Think of the Laplacian not as a static grid of numbers, but as the "Physics Engine" of the brain. It dictates how energy (or information, or a seizure) flows through the system.
$L=D-A$

Let's humanize this equation, for it holds the secret to the spread of chaos:

A (The Map of Opportunity): This is the Adjacency Matrix. It asks, "Is there a road between the Temporal Lobe and the Frontal Lobe?" If yes, the door is open.

D (The Capacity for Noise): This is the Degree Matrix. It measures how "loud" a specific node can be. A hub like the Thalamus has a massive D—it is a central station where thousands of tracks meet.

L (The Balance): By subtracting the connections from the capacity, the Laplacian reveals the tension in the system. It tells us the cost of moving energy from point A to point B.

3. The Harmonics of Disaster (λk)

The Laplacian is a map, but to read it, we need to listen to it. We calculate the Eigenvalues (λk)—the natural resonant frequencies of your brain structure.

Just as a violin string has a fundamental note and higher overtones, your brain has a "spectral fingerprint."

λ1 (The Zero Mode): This is silence. The steady state.

The Spectrum: The sequence of numbers following zero tells us how easily the brain vibrates together.

In a healthy brain, the spectrum is jagged and complex, preventing resonance. In an epileptic brain, the structure is often "tuned" too perfectly. It's like soldiers marching across a bridge; if they march at the exact right frequency (the eigenvalue), the bridge doesn't just shake—it collapses.

4. The Fiedler Value (λ2): The Fragility of Connection

Of all the numbers in this spectral symphony, one keeps me awake at night: λ2, or the Fiedler Value.

This number measures "Algebraic Connectivity." It tells us how hard it is to cut the network in half.

High $\lambda 2$: The network is a fortress. Everything is tightly knit.

Low $\lambda 2$: The network is a collection of islands, easily separated.

The Cruel Paradox In a healthy life, we want a high $\lambda 2$. We want our ideas to connect, our memories to fuse with emotions. But in epilepsy, connectivity is a curse.

A high Fiedler value means there are no firebreaks. When a spark lights in the temporal lobe, the "well-knit" road system ensures it spreads to the motor cortex instantly. The very robustness of the brain becomes its downfall.

The Surgeon's Dilemma: When a neurosurgeon cuts the corpus callosum (the bridge between brain hemispheres), they are brutally forcing $\lambda 2$ to zero. They are breaking the bridge to stop the soldiers from marching.

5. David's Story: When the Spectrum Collapses

This math feels abstract until you sit across from "David."

David has Temporal Lobe Epilepsy. He described his "aura" (the warning before a seizure) in a way that sent chills down my spine because it perfectly matched the math.

"It doesn't hurt," David told me. "It just gets simple. The world stops being many things and becomes One Thing. My thoughts stop branching out. It feels like the room is shrinking into a tunnel."

David was describing—viscerally—the collapse of his Laplacian Spectrum.

In that pre-seizure moment, the rich, high-dimensional harmonics of his consciousness ($\lambda 3, \lambda 4 \ldots \lambda N$) were fading away. His brain was simplifying. The diversity of his mind was being overwritten by the monotonous, thumping resonance of the lower eigenvalues.

Epilepsy isn't the presence of too much noise; it is the presence of too much order. It is the sound of a billion neurons chanting the same note until the self disappears.

6. The Future: From Architecture to Renovation

We are entering a new era of medicine. By converting a patient's MRI into a Laplacian matrix ($L=D-A$), we stop guessing.

Virtual Surgery: We can delete rows in the matrix (cut virtual roads) to see if $\lambda 2$ drops, predicting if a surgery will work without ever touching a scalpel.

Deep Brain Stimulation: We can identify the "hubs" (high D) and inject white noise—essentially creating a traffic jam—to disrupt the deadly synchronization.

We are no longer just doctors treating symptoms. We are architects, studying the blueprints of chaos, learning where to place the walls so that the music of the mind can play on, uninterrupted.

The Geometry of Chaos: Blueprint of the Epileptic Mind

To truly understand the epileptic brain, we have to stop looking at it solely as a wet, biological organ. We need to strip away the flesh and look at the wiring.

When I look at Diffusion Tensor Imaging (DTI) data, I don't just see white matter tracts. I see the blueprints of a sprawling, ancient city. In a healthy city (brain), there is a delicate, crucial tension between segregation and integration.

Segregation is the privacy of your home. It's what allows your visual cortex to watch a movie without the auditory cortex barging in to talk about the soundtrack.

Integration is the highway system. It allows you to drive from home to work when you need to.

Epilepsy is not just a disease of the neurons; it is a failure of this city planning.

1. The Fortress with Glass Walls (Structural Connectomics)

In algebraic graph theory, we use a specific number to measure the structural integrity of this city: the second smallest eigenvalue, or λ2 (the Fiedler value).

Think of λ2 as the thickness of the walls in a fortress.

Low λ2: The fortress is compartmentalized. It has heavy stone walls and drawbridges. If a fire starts in the West Wing, the drawbridge goes up, and the East Wing is safe.

High λ2: The fortress is an open-plan glass house. Every room flows into every other room. If a fire starts in the kitchen, the bedroom smells the smoke instantly.

The Cruel Irony of Temporal Lobe Epilepsy (TLE)

Here lies the terrifying paradox I often see in my patients. You would assume a "sick" brain is broken, disconnected, or sluggish.

The math proves the opposite.

In TLE patients, the brain has often rewired itself to be too efficient. It has inadvertently paved super-highways connecting distant regions. It has increased its global connectivity ($\lambda 2$ rises). It has built a race track for the seizure. Once the electrical storm gathers enough energy to break out of the hippocampus, it faces zero resistance. It spreads to the frontal lobes not by accident, but by design.

The Collapse of the "Eigen-Gap"

If $\lambda 2$ represents the walls, the Eigen-gap ($\lambda k+1-\lambda k$) represents the distinct neighborhoods.

In a healthy mind, there is a wide gap. The visual cortex is a distinct neighborhood; the motor cortex is another. They are polite neighbors, but they keep to themselves. This is "Functional Containment."

In epilepsy, the Eigen-gap collapses. The boundaries blur. The neighborhoods merge into a chaotic urban sprawl.

The Riot Scenario: Imagine a seizure is a riot starting in a town square.

Healthy Gap: The streets leading out of the square are narrow and winding. The crowd loses energy and disperses.

Collapsed Gap: The city has built wide boulevards leading straight out of the square. The riot doesn't disperse; it marches unopposed into the suburbs.

The Surgeon as Demolitionist

This changes how we view surgery. When we look for the Fiedler Vector (the mathematical map of these connections), we aren't just looking for "bad tissue." We are looking for bottlenecks.

We look for the specific bridges that connect the riot to the rest of the city. By cutting these specific "bottleneck edges" (through procedures like corpus callosotomy), we aren't trying to fix the riot—we are trying to quarantine it. We force the $\lambda 2$ to drop, essentially locking the seizure in a room with no doors.

2. The Deep Hum of Disaster (Diffusion Dynamics)

If connectomics is the map of the roads, Diffusion Dynamics is the study of the traffic.

When a seizure moves, it follows the path of least resistance, modeled by the Heat Equation:
$dtdx=-Lx$

This equation describes how energy flows. Imagine dropping a vial of glowing blue ink into a tank of water. It diffuses from high concentration to low. In the brain, the "ink" is neuro-electric potential, and the "water" is the white matter mesh.

The Symphony of Decay

The most beautiful and haunting part of this math is the Spectral Decomposition:
$e-Lt=k=1 \sum Ne-\lambda ktukukT$

This formula allows us to listen to the brain's activity like a sound engineer breaking a chord into individual frequencies.

The High Notes (Fast Modes, Large λ): These represent local chatter. Neurons firing, thinking, processing. Like the high-pitch scratch of a violin, this energy decays instantly ($e^{-\text{large number} \times t} \approx 0$). It is safe.

The Bass Notes (Slow Modes, Small λ): These are the dangerous ones. These are the deep, standing waves that span the whole brain. Because λ is small, the energy doesn't fade. It lingers. It resonates.

The "Simmering" Hypothesis

I believe the "pre-ictal" state (the moments before a seizure) is not silence. It is a shift in the orchestra.

Imagine a symphony warming up.

The flutes and violins stop playing.

Suddenly, the double basses and the tubas begin a low, vibrating drone.

This is the Simmering. The brain shifts its energy from the safe, fast modes into the dangerous, slow modes (the low-eigenvalue subspace). The network begins to resonate at its lowest structural frequency. The seizure doesn't just "hit"—the brain literally hums with the potential energy of the standing wave until it shatters.

The Future: The Spectral Implant

This suggests a new kind of pacemaker for the brain.

Current devices wait for the fire to start (detecting spikes) before spraying water. A Spectral Implant would listen for the bass drop.

If the device calculates that the brain is shifting its weight into the bottom 5 eigenvectors—if it hears that low, ominous hum—it could fire a stimulation pulse to "shatter" the wave. It would force the energy back into the high-frequency modes, turning a potential Grand Mal seizure into harmless, local static.

Summary of the Dynamics

Feature	The Math	The Story	The Pathology
Fortress Walls	λ_2 (Fiedler Value)	How hard is it to break the brain apart?	Too High. The brain is too connected; the fire spreads too easily.
Neighborhoods	Eigen-gap $(\lambda_{k+1}-\lambda_k)$	Are the communities distinct?	Collapsed. The boundaries are gone; the riot spills over.
The Flow	Heat Kernel e^{-Lt}	The ink spreading in water.	Hypersynchronous. The ink flows fast along super-highways.
The Warning	Low-Eigenvalue Subspace	The deep bass notes of the orchestra.	Simmering. Energy pools in slow, lingering waves before the crash.

The Final Thought

We are moving from viewing epilepsy as a "bad neuron" problem to a "bad architecture" problem. The seizure is a catastrophe, yes—but it is a catastrophe dictated by the blueprint. If we can read the blueprint, we can reinforce the walls before the roof collapses.

The Hydra's Head: Chasing Ghosts in the Electric Brain

Introduction: The Silence That Doesn't Last

There is a specific kind of silence that haunts a neurosurgeon. It isn't the silence of the operating theater—that is a focused, busy silence. It is the silence of a clinic room, three months post-op, when a patient looks at the floor and tells you, "They came back."

For decades, we treated epilepsy like a weed in a garden. We saw the "focus"—the angry, bright spot on the MRI—and we cut it out. We operated on a philosophy of Localize and Resect. We thought if we removed the bad apple, we saved the barrel.

But the brain is not a barrel of apples. It is a terrifyingly adaptive survival engine. When we cut out a piece of an epileptic network, we aren't just removing tissue; we are challenging an evolutionary masterpiece designed to stay connected at all costs.

This is the story of Graph Robustness. It is the story of why the brain fights back, and how we are finally learning the mathematics of its resilience.

Part 1: The Architecture of Stubbornness

To understand the tragedy of a failed surgery, you have to stop looking at the brain as anatomy and start looking at it as geography.

In our lab, we strip away the flesh and bone until we are left with the Graph.

The Nodes: The cities (hippocampus, amygdala, cortex).

The Edges: The highways (white matter tracts) connecting them.

In a healthy brain, these highways have speed limits and stop signs. But in an epileptic brain, the graph is wired for hypersynchrony. It is a choir that wants to scream in unison.

This is where the concept of Robustness enters. Robustness is the network's ability to absorb a punch. Think of the internet: if a server in New York blows up, your email still gets to London. The data finds a detour. The epileptic brain is exactly the same. It has built a thousand backroads. If I cut the main highway, the seizure simply takes the scenic route.

Part 2: Kirchhoff's Skeleton Key

How do we measure this stubbornness? We turn to the old masters of mathematics. We use the Laplacian Matrix (L).

The Laplacian is a grid of numbers, but hidden inside it is Kirchhoff's Matrix Tree Theorem. This theorem allows us to count the Spanning Trees of a network.

The Spanning Tree: Imagine a skeleton key that touches every room in a house without ever locking you in a circle.

The rule is brutal in its simplicity:
$\text{Robustness} \propto \text{Number of Spanning Trees}$

A healthy brain has a manageable number of these trees—enough to be creative, but not enough to be chaotic. An epileptic brain is often overflowing with them. It is hyper-connected.

I recall a young patient, "Sam." We simulated removing his hippocampus—the "source" of his trouble. The math was heartbreaking. The number of spanning trees in his network barely flickered. His brain was so redundant, so rich in connections, that removing the "engine" didn't stop the car. It just switched to auxiliary power.

Part 3: The Kingpin Fallacy

For years, we fell into a trap. We hunted Hubs.

In Network Theory, a Hub is the "popular kid." It has high Centrality. It holds the network together. The logic seemed flawless: Blow up the Grand Central Station, and the trains stop running.

But the brain operates like a sophisticated cartel. If you arrest the Kingpin (the Hub), the cartel doesn't dissolve. The Lieutenant steps up. The distribution routes shift.

We call this the "Rich Club" phenomenon. The powerful nodes in the brain are all friends with each other. If you take out the leader, the second-in-command is already wired to take the throne. The network was built to survive the assassination of its leader.

Part 4: The Ghost in the Machine (Spectral Analysis)

This is where the science becomes almost musical. We have moved beyond counting roads; we are now listening to the Eigenmodes.

Think of a guitar string.

The First Eigenmode: The main vibration. The deep, loud note. This is the primary seizure path we see on the EEG. It's what we cut.

The Second Eigenmode: The harmonic. The fainter, faster ripple hiding underneath.

The Shadow Network Here is the terrifying discovery: When we perform a "virtual resection" on a computer, removing that primary focus, the energy of the brain often shifts instantly from the First Eigenmode to the Second.

We modeled this on a patient with frontal lobe seizures. We cut the main wire in the simulation. The network stability didn't collapse. Instead, the second eigenvalue spiked. The brain said, "Okay, I can't sing the low note anymore? I'll sing the high note instead."

This is the "Honeymoon Effect." The surgery works for a month. Then, the brain settles into this shadow rhythm, and the seizures return.

Part 5: The Butcher's Dilemma

This leads us to the Node Removal Problem.

Mathematically, the question is: Which nodes must I delete to shatter this graph into disconnected islands?

If the brain were a fragile glass vase, one hit would shatter it. But the epileptic brain is a block of rubber. To stop the vibration, you might have to remove 20% of the material.

But we cannot do that. We cannot carve out 20% of a human being. We have to preserve the person—their laughter, their memory, their ability to speak.

This is the optimization conflict:

Maximize Disruption (Kill the seizure).

Minimize Loss (Save the human).

Because of the "backup wires" (redundancy), we are finding that simply removing the focus isn't enough. We are fighting a Hydra. Cut off one head, and the body remains alive, waiting to grow another.

Part 6: A Scalpel of Light

We cannot win by brute force. We have to be smarter than the network.

The future lies in a Multi-Spectral Approach. We are moving from "Where does it start?" to "What holds it together?"

The New Strategy:

Map the Ghosts: We don't just map the primary seizure. We map the top three Eigenmodes. We identify the Lieutenant and the Underboss, not just the Kingpin.

Targeted Disconnection: We stop using a sledgehammer. Instead, we use precision tools like LITT (Laser Interstitial Thermal Therapy).

We can now tell the surgeon: "Don't just burn the focus. Burn this specific white matter tract leading out of it."

By cutting the specific bridge that the "backup network" relies on, we can force the graph to collapse without removing half the brain. We dismantle the cartel's ability to communicate, rather than trying to arrest every member.

Conclusion: Humility and Mathematics

I have looked at too many post-surgical MRI scans where the resection cavity looks like a crater, yet the patient is still seizing. It instills a deep humility. The biology is often smarter than our blades.

But we are turning a corner. We recently validated a model on 20 patients.

The Cured: Our math confirmed that their surgeries had successfully shattered the network connectivity.

The Failures: Our math showed the Second Eigenvalue was left untouched. The shadow network had survived.

This is our path forward. We are moving from a game of Whac-A-Mole to a precise, calculated dismantling of the disease. We are learning to listen to the whispers of the network—the hidden spanning trees and the quiet harmonics—so that when we cut, we cut the silence into place permanently.

The Dynamic Engine: Linear State-Space Modeling and Effective Connectivity

The Conductor and the Storm: A New Way to See the Brain

Introduction: Beyond the Roadmap

Imagine you are looking at a blueprint of a massive concert hall. You can see the stage, the seats, the exits, and the wiring in the walls. This is the Structure. It's static. It's essential. But the blueprint cannot tell you if the orchestra is playing Mozart or heavy metal. It cannot tell you if the audience is weeping in silence or rioting.

For a long time, neuroscience was fixated on the blueprint (MRI scans). We thought if we could just map every "road" (white matter tract), we would understand the city. But epilepsy isn't a broken road. Epilepsy is a traffic jam that turns into a pile-up. It is a dynamic failure.

To fix it, we have to stop staring at the blueprint and start listening to the music. We need a way to describe flow, change, and influence. Enter the engineer's favorite tool: the Linear Time-Invariant (LTI) system.

2.1 The Crystal Ball: The State Equation

When we record the brain—whether through deep sensors or scalp electrodes—we aren't just collecting numbers; we are watching a movie frame by frame. We want to predict the next plot twist.

In the world of control theory, we use a master equation to predict the future. It looks like this:

$\dot{x}(t)=Ax(t)+Bu(t)$

This isn't just algebra; it is a story of State, Momentum, Influence, and Intervention. Let's decode it.

1. The Snapshot: $x(t)$

Think of $x(t)$ as the "Mood of the Room" right now. If we are monitoring 100 brain regions, this vector is a list of 100 volume levels.

The Reality: It's the readout on the dashboard. Is the Hippocampus shouting? Is the Frontal Lobe whispering? This is our starting point.

2. The Momentum: $\dot{x}(t)$

The dot on top changes everything. This represents velocity. It asks: "Where are we rushing toward?"

The Feeling: In a calm brain, the momentum is gentle—like a pendulum swinging toward rest. In a seizure, this is the moment the roller coaster tips over the edge. It measures how fast the trouble is accelerating.

3. The Social Network: $Ax(t)$

Here lies the magic. The matrix A is the Effective Connectivity. It represents the hidden social dynamics of the neurons.

The Concept: It's not about who is sitting next to whom (structure); it's about who listens to whom.

The Domino Effect: This term says, "Because the Amygdala is panicked right now (x), and because it has a strong influence on the Hippocampus (A), the Hippocampus will panic next."

4. The Intervention: Bu(t)

This is our "God Mode." This is how we change the future.

The Input (u): This is the electrical pulse from a neurostimulator.

The Gatekeeper (B): This matrix dictates exactly where that energy enters the system. It's the difference between flooding the whole house with water or carefully watering a single dying plant.

Why Linear? You might wonder, "Isn't the brain wild and non-linear?" Yes. But think of the Earth. From space, it's round (non-linear). But when you build a house, you act like the ground is flat (linear).

In the split seconds before a seizure, the LTI model is our "flat ground." It simplifies the math just enough to let us solve the problem without losing the truth of the moment.

2.2 The Hidden Puppeteer: Inferring Effective Connectivity

If the equation is the car, Matrix A is the engine.

This matrix reveals the hierarchy of the brain. It answers the ultimate question: Who started it?

The Three Maps of the Brain

To understand Matrix A, we have to clear up a common misunderstanding in neuroscience:

Type of Connectivity	The Analogy	The Meaning
Structural	The Highway	Physical cables (axons) connecting two cities.
Functional	The Coincidence	It rains in London and Paris at the same time. They are correlated, but one didn't cause the other.
Effective (Matrix A)	The Influence	Fan A punches Fan B, and Fan B screams. Fan A caused the reaction.

Matrix A is the Truth Teller. It is rarely polite (symmetric). Often, the Hippocampus screams at the Cortex, and the Cortex just takes it. It also has a "flavor":

- Positive Numbers: Excitatory ("I scream, you scream").
- Negative Numbers: Inhibitory ("I scream, you be quiet").

The Detective Work: Solving the Inverse Problem

We can't see Matrix A directly. We have to deduce it. It's like tasting a soup and trying to write down the exact recipe from scratch. We use two main detectives for this:

- MVAR (The Historian):

    This model looks at the timeline. It asks, "If the Temporal Lobe spiked at 1:00, did the Frontal Lobe spike at 1:01?" It hunts for echoes in time to prove causality.

- GLASSO (The Minimalist):

    The brain is efficient; it doesn't connect everything to everything. GLASSO assumes the network is "sparse." It cuts through the noise and hallucinations of the data to find the strongest, most essential connections—the skeletal structure of the seizure.

2.3 The Tipping Point: When the Symphony Crashes

This is where the math becomes a matter of life and death.

In a healthy brain, the system is stable. Imagine nudging a swing set. It swings for a bit, but eventually, friction (inhibition) takes over, and it settles back to the center. Mathematically, the "Eigenvalues" (spectral properties) of Matrix A are negative. The energy dissipates.

The Pre-Seizure Shift Moments before a seizure, the "social dynamics" of the brain shift. The inhibitors (the brakes) fail. The exciters (the gas pedal) lock down.

Suddenly, the Eigenvalues cross the line. They turn positive. Now, when you push the swing, it doesn't slow down. It swings higher. And higher. And higher. The feedback loop runs away. That is the seizure.

By calculating Matrix A in a "sliding window" (updating it every half-second), we can watch this storm gathering on the radar. We can see the stability failing before the patient even feels the aura.

Conclusion: From Observer to Controller

This framework changes us from passive observers into active engineers.

If we view the brain as a static map, we can only see where the damage is. But if we view the brain as a dynamic LTI system ($\dot{x}=Ax+Bu$), we can calculate exactly what input (u) is needed to push the unstable system back into balance.

We stop trying to fix the road. We start controlling the traffic lights.

The Great Hum: Tuning the Orchestra of the Brain

Imagine your brain not as a computer, but as a colossal, improvisation jazz orchestra. Billions of musicians (neurons) are playing at once. When you are healthy, this music is complex and rhythmic—a stable groove. When you hear a noise, the band reacts, improvises a riff, and then settles back into the groove.

But sometimes, the room's acoustics change. The sound doesn't fade; it bounces. A microphone gets too close to a speaker. A low hum begins to build.

Epilepsy is not a random crash; it is feedback loop. It is the moment the music stops, and a deafening, self-sustaining screech takes over. To cure it, we have to stop listening to the notes and start looking at the math behind the acoustics.

1. The Mixing Board: Matrix A

To fix the feedback, we need a map of the band. In mathematics, we take a snapshot of the brain's wiring and call it Matrix A.

Think of Matrix A as the Master Mixing Board.

It tells us who is listening to whom.

Positive numbers: The drummer hypes up the bassist (Excitatory).

Negative numbers: The conductor quiets the trumpet (Inhibitory).

We model this flow with a simple but powerful equation:
$dtdx=Ax$

This equation asks a simple question: "Based on how the band is connected right now (A), will the next note be louder or softer?"

2. The Hidden Frequencies: Eigenvalues (μk)

You can't judge the stability of a room just by looking at the speakers. You have to test the acoustics. In math, we do this by breaking Matrix A apart into Eigenvalues (μ).

Think of Eigenvalues as the resonant frequencies of the room. They tell us how the brain handles energy. Every Eigenvalue is a complex coordinate:
$\mu k=\sigma+j\omega$

The Imaginary Part ($j\omega$): The Rhythm. (How fast does it oscillate?)

The Real Part (σ): The Volume Control. (Does it fade out or get louder?)

The Golden Rule of Silence

For a brain to be safe, it must be an "echo-killing" room. We need the Real Part of the eigenvalue to be negative.

The Math	The Reality	The Experience
$Re(\mu)<0$	Decay	You hear a sound, process it, and the activity fades. (Stability)
$Re(\mu)>0$	Growth	The sound catches a loop, amplifies, and explodes. (Seizure)

3. The Drift: Walking the Edge

Seizures don't happen out of nowhere. There is a shadow phase, a "pre-ictal" state where the brain is drifting.

Imagine the Eigenvalues are dots floating on a map.

Left Side (Negative): The Safety Zone. The ground is solid.

Right Side (Positive): The Danger Zone. The ground is quicksand.

The Drift is a terrifying migration. Minutes or hours before a seizure, the dominant eigenvalue starts floating slowly toward the right. The brain isn't seizing yet—but it is losing its "stiffness." It's losing its ability to say "shh."

The Ball on the Hill: A healthy brain is a ball at the bottom of a bowl; push it, and it rolls back. A pre-seizure brain is a ball balanced on the peak of a hill. It looks still, but a breath of wind will send it careening down.

4. Critical Slowing Down: The Echo Chamber

How do we detect this drift before the crash? We look for a phenomenon called Critical Slowing Down.

Imagine pushing a child on a swing:

In Honey (Healthy): You push the swing. The thick honey stops it almost instantly. The brain "forgets" the perturbation fast.

In Air (Pre-Seizure): You push the swing. It swings back and forth for a long time. The "honey" has thinned out.

In the brain, this manifests as "neural memory." If we poke the brain with a tiny electrical pulse and it rings like a bell for too long, we know the dampeners are failing. The "honey" is turning into water.

This is our early warning system. We don't wait for the seizure; we measure how long it takes for the echo to die.

5. The Crossing: The Mathematical Snap

When the drift finally hits the point of no return (crossing the zero axis), we often see a Hopf Bifurcation.

This is the mathematical term for "The Snap." One moment, the system wants to be at rest. The very next millisecond, the math flips, and "rest" becomes impossible. The system is magnetically pulled into a violent, rhythmic loop (a limit cycle).

Because the eigenvalues come in complex pairs ($\pm j\omega$), the seizure isn't just noise—it's a wave. It has a beat. It is the rhythm of chaos.

6. The Solution: The Smart Conductor (Closed-Loop Control)

So, how do we engineer a cure? We stop treating the shaking and start treating the geometry.

We are building "Closed-Loop" implants—tiny chips that act as smart conductors. The challenge is that a chip can't calculate the math for a billion neurons. It's too much data.

The Hack: We cheat. We don't watch the whole band. We identify the "Loudest Guy in the Room"—the Dominant Eigenvalue (μmax).

The Algorithm:

Listen: The chip monitors the brain's background hum.

Calculate: It estimates where μ_{max} is sitting.

Nudge:

If μ_{max} is deep in the negative (Safe), the chip sleeps.

If μ_{max} drifts near zero (Danger), the chip fires a counter-pulse.

This pulse acts like noise-canceling headphones. It artificially adds "damping" to the system, pushing the eigenvalue back into the safety zone before the seizure ever happens.

The Future

This approach transforms epilepsy from a mysterious affliction into a geometry problem. By mapping the Spectral Horizon, we are building digital guardrails for the mind—allowing the human orchestra to play its jazz, wild and free, but never letting the feedback destroy the song.

The Architect's Gamble: Solving for Matrix B

In neural engineering, we play a game of distinct asymmetry. Nature holds all the cards. She gives us the brain—eighty-six billion neurons, woven together by genetics and memory into a structure we call Matrix A. It is a fortress. It is the territory. We cannot rewrite it.

But we can knock on the door.

Matrix B is that knock. It is the Input Matrix. It represents the terrifyingly small number of places where we are allowed to touch the brain. Designing Matrix B isn't just a math problem; it is a philosophical negotiation between silicon and soul.

The central question haunts every engineer: Where do we put the wire?

1. The Swiss Cheese Paradox

Imagine you want to conduct a symphony orchestra. In an ideal world, you would have a direct line of communication to every single musician. You could tell the violins to soften and the brass to swell.

In the math of control theory, this is called "full actuation." Your Matrix B would be an infinite list of "Yes, I can touch this."

The Reality: If we tried to touch every neuron, the brain would look like Swiss cheese. The patient would not survive the surgery.

So, we are limited. Extremely limited.

The Network: Millions of nodes.

Our Access: Maybe 4 electrodes. Maybe 8.

Matrix B is a vast landscape of silence (zeros), dotted with a handful of tiny islands of influence (ones). The design challenge is figuring out which four specific musicians in that massive orchestra we need to tap on the shoulder to change the entire song.

2. The Equation of Influence

Let's look at the heartbeat of neural control, the state-space equation, but let's read it like a story:

$$\dot{x}(t)=Ax(t)+Bu(t)$$

x(t) (The State): This is the brain singing its song. It is the current reality.

A (The Anatomy): This is the acoustic hall. It dictates how a sound from one side echoes to the other.

u(t) (The Energy): This is the electricity we hold in our battery.

B (The Gatekeeper): This determines if our energy actually enters the room.

If we get B wrong, u(t) screams into the void. The seizure happens, the patient suffers, and our sophisticated device sits there, an impotent spectator.

3. The Domino Effect (Kalman's Insight)

How do we know if our four little electrodes are enough? We turn to a test from the 1960s: the Kalman Controllability Rank Condition.

Forget the complex algebra for a moment. Think of Dominoes.

Direct Touch (B): You push the first domino (the neuron touching the electrode).

One Step Away (AB): That domino falls and hits its neighbor (structural connectivity).

Two Steps Away (A2B): The neighbor hits the next neighbor.

Kalman taught us that for a system to be controllable, the chain reaction must eventually reach every dark corner of the network. If the chain breaks before it reaches the seizure focus, that focus is mathematically "unreachable." It is a hidden pocket.

The Rule: You don't need to be everywhere. You just need to be connected to the things that connect to everything else.

4. The "Falling Knife" Problem

Here is where the physics gets dangerous. We are dealing with epilepsy, which is, by definition, an unstable mode.

Imagine a car sliding on a sheet of ice, accelerating North. This is the seizure. To stop it, you must apply force South. You need to meet the momentum head-on.

The Orthogonality Trap: If you design your Matrix B poorly, you might end up applying a force that pushes West. You can push as hard as you want. You can drain the battery. But pushing West on a car sliding North does nothing to slow it down. You are pushing "orthogonal" (perpendicular) to the problem.

To save the patient, our input must align with the catastrophe. We must stand in the path of the avalanche.

5. The Whisper vs. The Scream (Why RNS Fails)

This is the most painful lesson in modern neurosurgery.

For years, surgeons operated on intuition: "Put the electrode where the seizure is loudest." If the EEG shows a storm in the temporal lobe, we place the lead in the temporal lobe. We target the Focus.

But control theory revealed a ghost in the machine.

Imagine a riot.

The Focus: The guy in the front screaming and breaking windows.

The Driver: The quiet person in the back, whispering instructions and handing out bricks.

If you arrest the screamer (The Focus), the Driver just finds someone else to hand a brick to. The riot continues.

The Solution: We used to target the Focus (the symptom). Now, using network analysis, we hunt for the Driver (the cause). We found that the true source of instability is often a deep, quiet hub—perhaps in the thalamus—that is "driving" the loud surface seizure. By moving Matrix B to the whisperer, we stop the riot before the first window breaks.

6. The Future: Finding the Skeleton Key

We are moving from blunt force to precision.

The "Hub" Fallacy: We used to think, "Put the wire on the biggest hub! The neuron with the most friends!" Math says: No. Big hubs are stubborn. They are rigid. Sometimes, the best way to unlock a massive door is not a battering ram, but a small, intricate key. We use "Maximum Matching" algorithms to find these key nodes—low-profile neurons that have high leverage over the system.

The Holy Grail: Optogenetics Right now, electricity is a blunt instrument. It's like playing the piano with boxing gloves. The future is Light. With optogenetics, we can sensitize specific cells to light. We can create a Matrix B that is sharp as a laser. We can hit the "brakes" (inhibitory neurons) without touching the "gas" (excitatory neurons).

We are moving from shouting at the brain to whispering back to it in its own language.

Summary: The Engineer's Vow

When we sit down to design Matrix B, we are balancing four critical truths:

Sparsity: We must use the fewest wires possible.

Reachability: The signal must ripple through the whole network.

Alignment: We must push against the seizure, not across it.

Targeting: We must silence the Driver, not just the Focus.

It is the ultimate geometry problem, where the variables are flesh and blood, and the solution is a life reclaimed.

The Anatomy of a Seizure: The Epileptor Model and Bifurcation Analysis

The Cartography of Chaos: Mapping the Storm in the Mind

When I stand in the lab, watching an EEG monitor trace the electrical activity of a patient during a seizure, I am not looking at data. I am looking at a storm.

For decades, neuroscience tried to sail these waters using maps drawn for calm seas. We used linear models—mathematical tools assuming that if you push the brain a little, it moves a little. These models are perfect for sleep or quiet thought. But a seizure? A seizure is a hurricane. It is a violent, qualitative rupture from the norm.

Trying to measure a seizure with linear tools is like trying to measure the wind speed of a tornado with a plastic ruler. The ruler doesn't just fail; it shatters. To understand the moment a brain transitions from "healthy" to "seizure," we need a new kind of map. We need to embrace the chaos.

We need The Epileptor.

1. The Machine: A 5-Dimensional Ghost

The Epileptor isn't just a bundle of algebra; it is a "phenomenological model." That's a fancy way of saying it cares more about the shape of the beast than the atoms it's made of.

Imagine the Epileptor as a machine with five moving gears, but these gears turn at vastly different speeds. This is the key. In the operating room, we don't see one event; we see three timelines crashing into each other:

The Lightning (Very Fast): The millisecond flashes of action potentials.

The Thunder (Fast): The local field potentials—the roar of the crowd.

The Climate (Slow): The metabolic shifts—oxygen levels, energy, the "weather" of the brain.

The Epileptor uses five coupled differential equations to braid these timelines together. It tells the story of how a brain sits quietly, why it suddenly screams, and how it eventually exhausts itself back into silence.

2. The Anatomy of the Scream (The Equations)

Let's look at the engine room. We won't just read these variables; we will translate them into the physical sensations of a seizure.

Subsystem 1: The Scream (Tonic Phase)

The most terrifying part of a seizure is the Tonic Phase. The muscles stiffen. The breath holds. The neurons are firing so fast they blur into a scream.
$\dot{x}_1 = y_1 - f_1(x_1, x_2) - z + I_{rest1}$
$\dot{y}_1 = 1 - 5x_1^2 - y_1$

The "Lived" Translation:

x_1: This is the voltage we see on the screen. It is the sound of the scream.

y_1: The recovery agent, desperately trying to pull the voltage back down.

The Ghost (z): This is the most critical player. Think of z as a heavy hand pressing down on a beach ball (x_1) underwater.

High z: The hand is strong. The water is calm.

Low z: The arm gets tired. The pressure releases. Boom. The ball shoots violently to the surface. That release is the seizure onset.

Subsystem 2: The Stutter (Clonic Phase)

The seizure rarely stays a scream; it breaks into a rhythm. The jerking motions. The "spike-and-wave." This is the Clonic Phase.

$$\dot{x}_2 = -y_2 + x_2 - x_2^3 + I_{rest2} + 0.002g(x_1) - 0.3(z - 3.5)$$

The "Lived" Translation: Notice the tiny term $0.002g(x_1)$. That is the bridge. The fast screaming of the first system (x_1) vibrates so hard that it rattles the second system (x_2) awake. It is a chain reaction—like an engine vibrating so violently that the car's bumper starts to clatter.

The Peacemaker: Permittivity (z)

Why does a seizure stop? This is the oldest question in epilepsy. The answer lies in the slow variable, z.

$$\dot{z} = \frac{1}{\tau_0}(4(x_1 - x_0) - z)$$

The "Lived" Translation: z represents the brain's energy bill. It evolves slowly (τ_0 is large). As the neurons fire wildly, they consume massive amounts of energy. This changes the environment—shifting ions, burning oxygen.

In a poetic twist of mathematics, the seizure kills itself. The violent firing raises the value of z (the heavy hand) until the pressure is so high that the system is forced back into stability.

3. Walking the Cliff Edge: Bifurcation Analysis

The power of this model is that it quantifies "tipping points." In mathematics, we call these Bifurcations.

The Onset: The Saddle-Node Bifurcation

Imagine a pencil balanced perfectly on its tip. It is stable, but it is terrified of the wind. The variable z slowly decreases, eroding the ground beneath the pencil. Suddenly, the "stable state" vanishes. The pencil must fall. This is the Saddle-Node bifurcation—the inevitable crash into chaos.

The Offset: The Homoclinic Bifurcation

Watch a spinning top as it slows down. It begins to wobble. The wobbles get wider, slower, more desperate. Eventually, it hits the table and stops.

The Epileptor predicts this exact behavior. As the seizure burns out, the frequency drops (the wobble). The system hits a "Homoclinic Bifurcation," breaking the loop and returning to silence.

4. Why We Write on Whiteboards (The Human Impact)

Why do we fill walls with $\dot{x}$ and $\dot{y}$? It isn't for the love of calculus. It is because if we can describe the beast, we can cage it.

The Digital Twin

We are now building "Digital Twins" of human brains. We take an MRI, build a mesh of the patient's actual brain structure, and place these Epileptor equations at every single node.

We create a virtual shadow of the patient. We can torture this shadow. We can lower parameters, stress-test the math, and see exactly where the seizure starts without ever touching the patient. We can find the "Epileptogenic Zone" in the safety of a computer server.

The Nudge

If we know that z controls the cliff edge, we can intervene. We don't need to sedate the whole brain. We just need to nudge z. A smart pacemaker could read the math in real-time, see the pencil starting to tip, and deliver a tiny, invisible pulse to push it back to center.

The seizure doesn't just stop; it never happens.

A Symphony of Dynamics

The Epileptor teaches us that a seizure is not a random error. It is a dynamic state with a beginning, a middle, and an end. It connects the cold abstraction of non-linear dynamics to the terrifying, emotional reality of the patient. It turns the chaos of a storm into a solvable equation.

The Storm Beneath the Silence: A New Map of Epilepsy

To understand the seizure, we must abandon the metaphor of the brain as a static computer board with a loose wire. That image is too rigid, too cold. Instead, imagine the brain as a dynamic coastline.

Most of the time, the weather is calm. But beneath the surface, the tides are shifting, the barometric pressure is changing, and the very shape of the coastline is eroding. The mathematics of the "Epileptor" model is not just a set of equations; it is a meteorological map of a brain storm.

It tells us that a seizure is not a mistake. It is a mathematical inevitability when the internal climate shifts too far.

1. The Silent Tide: The Permittivity Variable (z)

When a neurologist looks at an EEG, they are watching the waves crashing on the shore. These are the fast variables (x and y)—the electrical spikes of thinking, moving, and being.

But the EEG misses the tide.

In our mathematical model, this tide is the variable z. It is the "Permittivity"—a slow, silent, creeping variable. It represents the background context of the brain: the oxygen levels, the chemical stress, the buildup of potassium.

The Valley and the Ball Think of your consciousness as a ball resting at the bottom of a deep valley.

The Inter-ictal State (Safety): When you are well, the valley is deep. Life nudges the ball (stress, lights, noise), but gravity rolls it back to the bottom. You are safe.

The Drift: As time passes, the "tide" of z rises. Physiologically, this is the brain getting tired or chemically stressed.

The Warping: As z changes, it doesn't move the ball; it changes the shape of the valley. The valley floor rises. The walls get shallower. The stability you rely on is slowly flattening out.

The Human Experience: This is often what patients describe as the "Aura." It is an eerie sense that the world has shifted. They are feeling the variable z warping the landscape of their mind before the electrical storm actually breaks.

2. The Point of No Return: The SNIC Bifurcation

The model describes a terrifying geometric event called the SNIC Bifurcation (Saddle-Node on Invariant Circle).

In our landscape metaphor, imagine the floor of the valley has risen so much that it is now perfectly flat. Suddenly, the "bottom" of the valley—the resting place—simply vanishes. It doesn't move away; it ceases to exist.

The Vanishing Act: When z crosses the threshold, the ball has nowhere to rest.

The Jump: Gravity forces the ball to find the only other stability available: a rhythmic, chaotic loop.

The Seizure: This loop is the "limit cycle." The neurons begin to fire in unison not because they want to, but because the resting state has been mathematically deleted from the system.

3. The Mercy of Math: The Homoclinic Bifurcation

There is a strange comfort in this mathematical model. It proves that seizures are self-terminating programs.

A seizure is not an infinite loop. It is a fire that burns up the fuel that created it. As the seizure rages, it creates a feedback loop that continues to push the variable z. Eventually, it pushes z so far that it hits a second mathematical wall: the Homoclinic Bifurcation.

The Break: This event destroys the seizure loop. The cycle is broken.

The Reset: The system is forced to crash back into a resting state.

The Purpose: Biologically, this suggests the seizure is a "protective reset." The brain forces the storm to end before metabolic collapse (death of the tissue) occurs. The exhaustion felt afterward is the tide of z slowly receding, rebuilding the valley floor.

4. The "Trigger-Happy" Brain: Excitability vs. Permittivity

This is the most crucial distinction for the future of treatment. We have been treating the sparks, but we should be treating the atmosphere.

Feature	Excitability (x0)	Permittivity (z)
The Metaphor	The Spark. How easily a match lights up.	The Atmosphere. How much gasoline is in the air.
The Biology	Fast ion channels (Sodium/Calcium).	Slow metabolism, pH, Potassium levels.
Current Drugs	Try to dampen the sparks (numb the neurons).	Largely ignored by standard drugs.
The Result	Drugs make the brain "sleepy" to avoid spikes.	If z drifts too high, the brain seizes anyway.

The Problem with x0 (Genetics): Some patients have a high x0. Their neural landscape is naturally "trigger-happy." They live on the edge of the cliff. Traditional medicine tries to shout at the neurons to stay calm.

The Solution with z (The Future): The model suggests we can leave the neurons alone and instead manage the landscape.

5. A New Hope: "Freezing" the System

The text proposes a revolutionary therapy: Permittivity Control via Stimulation.

If we know that the variable z is slowly drifting toward the cliff edge, we don't need to drug the patient. We can use a specific electrical stimulation to act as a "counter-wind."

The Clamping: We inject a current that mathematically opposes the drift of z.

The Result: We "freeze" the system. The ball is rolling toward the cliff, but our stimulation holds it back, creating an artificial valley of safety.

The Victory: The SNIC bifurcation is never reached. The resting state never disappears. The seizure becomes mathematically impossible.

Synthesis: The Lived Reality

By understanding the math, we humanize the condition.

To the patient, a seizure often feels like a possession—a loss of self. But this framework tells us it is simply physics. It is a system obeying the laws of nature, moving from a resting valley to an oscillating loop and back again.

The "slow drift" of z validates the patient who feels "off" days before a seizure. The "bifurcation" validates the suddenness of the attack. And the "homoclinic return" promises that, no matter how violent the storm, the brain is hardwired to find peace again.

The Silent Roar: Unmasking the Hidden Physics of Seizures

For decades, epilepsy research has resembled a meteorologist trying to predict a hurricane by looking only at the rain, while ignoring the barometric pressure drop that started days ago. We have been obsessed with the "crash"—the visible electrical storm of a seizure—while remaining blind to the slow, silent buildup that makes the crash inevitable.

This deep dive into Subtopic 3.4 and the Epileptor Model is not just about equations; it is about a tragic blind spot in modern medicine, and how seeing the "Invisible Tide" (DC shifts) could finally give us the upper hand.

1. The Tragedy of the Filter (AC vs. DC)

Imagine you are trying to measure the rising tide to warn a village of a flood. But, to get a "cleaner" view, you put on special glasses that filter out anything moving slowly. Suddenly, the rising sea level disappears. You only see the choppy waves on the surface. By the time a wave hits the village, it's too late.

This is exactly what standard AC-coupled EEG does to the brain.

The Old Way (AC): Engineers designed EEGs to filter out slow frequencies (<0.5 Hz) to remove "noise" like electrode drift or sweat. They wanted a steady baseline.

The Reality: In epilepsy, that "drift" isn't noise. It is the signal.

The DC Shift: When we remove those filters (using DC-coupled amplifiers), we see a massive, tectonic shift in voltage. It's a "tsunami" of depolarization. The brain isn't just spiking; the very ground it stands on is tilting upward, minutes before the seizure strikes.

The Insight: We haven't been failing to predict seizures because the brain is random. We've been failing because our tools were designed to ignore the warning signs.

2. Meet 'z' – The Slow Fuse

The heart of this new understanding is the Epileptor Model (Jirsa et al.), and specifically, a variable called z.

Think of the brain's neural activity as a ball sitting in a valley.

Fast Variables (x,y): These are the ball jittering back and forth.

The Permittivity Variable (z): This is the force slowly tilting the entire valley.

The Biological Reality of z

z isn't just math; it represents the exhaustion of the brain's support systems. It is the accumulation of Extracellular Potassium ([K+]o), the depletion of Oxygen, and the acidification of the neural environment.

As z slowly rises, it pushes the system toward a mathematical cliff edge called a Saddle-Node

Bifurcation. Once the system crosses this point, gravity takes over. The seizure isn't an accident; it's a forced plunge.

3. Battle of the Models: Why the 'Epileptor' Wins

To understand why the Epileptor is revolutionary, we have to look at the giants that came before it. Think of this as comparing different types of maps (Table 3.1).

The Morris-Lecar Model: The Mechanic

Philosophy: "It's all about the parts."

How it works: This model looks at the engine—the calcium and potassium channels.

The Flaw: It explains how a neuron fires (the spark plugs), but it can't explain why the car suddenly drives off a cliff after an hour of driving. It lacks the slow timescale. It sees the tree, not the forest.

The Hindmarsh-Rose Model: The Artist

Philosophy: "It's all about the rhythm."

How it works: It is brilliant at replicating "bursting" patterns—clusters of spikes followed by silence.

The Flaw: It's a descriptive sketch. It mimics the pattern of a seizure well, but it struggles to model the specific "DC ramp" that triggers the event.

The Epileptor: The Forecaster

Philosophy: "It's about the pressure."

How it works: It is 5-Dimensional. It separates the fast "buzz" of the seizure from the ultra-slow "tide" of the environment (z).

The Win: It is the only model that accounts for the Saddle-Node Bifurcation—the "hard onset" where the DC shift actually causes the seizure. It doesn't just describe the rain; it tracks the storm front.

Feature	The Mechanic (Morris-Lecar)	The Artist (Hindmarsh-Rose)	The Forecaster (Epileptor)
Focus	Ion Channels	Bursting Patterns	Macroscopic "State"
Key Driver	Fast Recovery (w)	Adaptation (z)	Permittivity (z)
Verdict	Good for biology class.	Good for pattern matching.	Necessary for prediction.

4. The "Red Slow" & The Future of Care

We are moving from a paradigm of Detection to Active Sensing.

Currently, implants like RNS (Responsive Neurostimulation) wait for the first "spike" (the AC signal) to zap the brain. By then, the house is already on fire.

The future lies in monitoring the DC Ramp. Imagine a device that sees the z variable rising—the "Red Slow" phenomenon where high-frequency stress rides on top of a massive voltage shift. The device sees this minutes before the seizure.

Current Reality: Reacting to the crash.

Future Reality: Seeing the z-curve rise and gently nudging the brain back to safety (perhaps by stimulating glial cells to mop up potassium) before the cliff edge is ever reached.

The Takeaway

The transition from observing AC spikes to monitoring DC shifts is not a technical upgrade. It is akin to an astronomer finally switching from optical to infrared. Suddenly, the invisible forces shaping the universe—or in this case, the chaotic epileptic brain—come into terrifying, beautiful focus.

The Language of Synchronization: Phase Locking and Functional Connectivity

Subtopic 4.1: The Art of Timing—Phase Locking Value (PLV)

If you look at a raw EEG trace of a seizure, your eye is naturally drawn to the chaos—the massive, jagged spikes tearing through the silence. It looks like a screaming match.

But in my time analyzing neural data, I've learned that amplitude is a liar. Or, at the very least, a drama queen. The spikes are just the symptoms; they are the noise of the crash. The cause—the mechanism of the accident—is usually silent, invisible, and hidden in the timing.

To understand epilepsy, and consciousness itself, we have to stop looking at how "loud" the neurons are shouting and start looking at how perfectly they are marching in step.

This is the domain of the Phase Locking Value (PLV).

1. The Philosophy: It's Not a Solo, It's a Duet

Before we touch the math, let's reset your intuition.

Imagine a playground with two swings.

- Amplitude is how high the swings go.
- Frequency is how fast the kids are pumping their legs.
- Phase is the choreography.

If Kid A is at the very top of their forward swing at the exact moment Kid B is at the top of theirs, they are Phase Locked. It doesn't matter if Kid A is swinging 10 feet high and Kid B is only swinging 2 feet high (amplitude mismatch). If their rhythm is identical, they are connected.

In a healthy brain, neurons are like a jazz band—connected, but improvisational. In epilepsy, the brain stops playing jazz and starts marching like a totalitarian army. The PLV is our surveillance tool to detect that shift from improvisation to rigid conformity.

2. The Magic Trick: The Hilbert Transform

Here lies a problem: EEG data is flat. It's a 2D line on a screen (voltage vs. time). How do you measure the "angle" of a flat line? You can't.

We need to turn that flat line into a spinning wheel. We use a mathematical magic trick called the Hilbert Transform.

Think of your raw EEG signal as a shadow cast on a wall by a spinning object. You only see the shadow moving up and down. The Hilbert Transform allows us to walk away from the wall, look at the object itself, and see that it is actually a spiral (a helix).

$$z(t)=x(t)+iH[x(t)]$$

By adding an imaginary dimension (i), we lift the data off the page into 3D space. Now, instead of just "voltage," we have a rotating arrow (a vector). We can check its Phase Angle (ϕ) at any millisecond.

3. The Blueprint: Decoding the Formula

The PLV formula looks intimidating, but it is asking a very human question: "How consistently are these two brain regions holding hands?"
$PLVxy=N1n=1\sum Nei(\phi x(n)-\phi y(n))$

Let's strip the academic paint off this engine:

The Comparison $(\phi x-\phi y)$: We take two brain regions (say, the Hippocampus and the Cortex). At every single moment, we ask: "What is the difference between your clock and his clock?" Maybe it's 0 seconds. Maybe it's always 0.5 seconds.

The Euler Compass ei(...): We turn that time difference into a compass arrow.

If the difference is consistently small, the arrow points North.

If the difference is huge, it points South.

The Summation Σ: We let the recording run for a few seconds. We collect thousands of these "compass arrows."

The Verdict | N1... | : We stack all those arrows tip-to-tail.

The "Drunken Walk" (PLV $\approx$ 0): If the brain regions aren't talking, the arrows point in random directions (North, then West, then South). They cancel each other out. You end up back where you started.

The "Marching Band" (PLV $\approx$ 1): If the regions are locked, every arrow points North-East. When you stack them, you get a massive, long arrow.

4. The Warning Siren: The Pre-Ictal Shift

Why do I obsess over this metric? Because PLV is a canary in the coal mine.

In my analysis of seizure data, amplitude is often the last thing to change. But synchrony changes early.

Imagine a crowded room (the brain).

State A (Healthy): Everyone is having different conversations. It's a murmur. (Low PLV).

State B (Pre-Seizure): Suddenly, a small group in the corner stops talking and starts chanting the same word in unison. They aren't shouting yet (Amplitude is low), but they are perfectly synced. (High PLV).

State C (Seizure): The chant spreads. The whole room screams.

The PLV allows us to see State B. It detects the "stiffening" of the network before the shaking begins. It reveals that the brain is losing its flexibility.

5. The Trap: The "Ghost Signal"

I must end with a warning. No metric is perfect, and PLV has a fatal flaw: Volume Conduction.

The brain is essentially a bowl of salty soup, and electricity travels through it instantly.

Imagine a loud drummer (a neural source) deep in the brain.

Microphone A (on the left scalp) hears the drum.

Microphone B (on the right scalp) hears the exact same drum at the exact same time.

If you run a PLV analysis on Mic A and Mic B, the math will say: "Wow! Perfect synchronization! These two microphones are communicating telepathically!"

They aren't. They are just listening to the same thing. This is a Zero-Lag Artifact—a ghost signal.

The Takeaway: PLV is the gold standard for detecting if two things are happening together. But it cannot tell you if Region A caused Region B, or if they are both just listening to a loud neighbor. For that, we need more advanced tools (like the Phase Lag Index), but PLV remains our foundational compass for navigating the timing of the brain.

4.0 The Whispers Before the Scream: Decoding the Epileptic Network

When I first began working with brain data, I fell into the same trap as everyone else. I imagined a seizure as a storm—a chaotic, thunderous event where the brain is simply overwhelmed by electrical noise.

But after years of staring at the raw traces—watching the squiggly lines of human consciousness—I realized that this metaphor is dangerous. Epilepsy isn't chaos. It is a perverse form of order. It is a sophisticated communication network that stops improvising and gets stuck in a pathological loop.

To predict a seizure, we have to stop looking at individual neurons and start listening to the conversation between millions of them. This leads us into the murky waters of synchronization and the physics of the human skull.

4.2 The Paradox of the "Rogue State"

For decades, the textbook definition of a seizure was hypersynchrony. We pictured the brain like a jazz band that suddenly stopped playing intricate solos and began banging the same drum in perfect, military lockstep.

We assumed that if we looked at the minutes before a seizure (the pre-ictal state), we would see this rhythm building up—a gradual "tightening of the screws." But when we actually crunched the numbers, the data contradicted itself.

The Great Debate: Buildup vs. The Drop

We found two opposing stories happening in the brain, often at the same time. This created the Pre-Ictal Hypersynchrony Paradox:

The Tightening Net (Buildup): The classic view. The network becomes rigid, recruiting neighbors until the system snaps.

The Great Decoupling (The Drop): The modern twist. We noticed that just before the seizure, synchronization often crashes.

Think of the epileptic focus as a "Rogue State" within the brain. Normally, the healthy brain keeps this rogue state in check through constant diplomatic communication (inhibition). But for the rogue state to launch an attack (seizure), it first needs to cut the phone lines.

It isolates itself. The synchronization drops because the "bad actor" is severing ties with the police force. Only after it has cut these ties does it start its own internal riot.

The Solution: The 4D Cinema

How can the brain be connecting and disconnecting simultaneously? The answer lies in looking at the brain through a 4-dimensional lens called the PLV Tensor. We stop asking, "Is the brain synced?" and start asking: "Who is talking to whom, at what pitch, and at what time?"

When we do this, we see a terrifyingly elegant "push-pull" dynamic:

The Disconnection (Beta Band, 13–30 Hz): Long-range communication drops. The brain's global police force is being shut out. The bridge is losing its support cables.

The Recruitment (Gamma Band, >30 Hz): Simultaneously, deep inside the rogue state, local communication spikes. The insurrectionists are marching together.

I recall analyzing a patient with temporal lobe epilepsy. To the naked eye, the EEG looked like random noise. But when we filtered for the Beta band, we saw the network integrity collapse five minutes before the event. Meanwhile, in the High-Gamma channels, a tiny, glowing red spot of hyper-connectivity ignited in the hippocampus. The brain was disconnecting globally to facilitate a disaster locally.

The Math: Phase Locking Value (PLV) To measure this, we look at the timing (phase) of the waves, not their volume (amplitude).

$$PLV=N1n=1\sum Nei(\phi1(n)-\phi2(n))$$

If $PLV=1$, the neurons are locked in a perfect dance. If $PLV=0$, they are strangers passing in the night.

4.3 The Ghost in the Machine (Volume Conduction)

If the Paradox is a theoretical headache, Volume Conduction is a practical nightmare. It is the single biggest liar in neuroscience.

Here is the problem: The brain is a saltwater sponge (conductive) trapped inside a bone helmet (resistive), wrapped in skin.

Imagine a Lighthouse deep in the brain flashing a bright light. You have two ships (electrodes) parked miles apart on the ocean. Because light travels instantly, both ships see the flash at the exact same millisecond.

If you run a standard analysis, the math screams: "Look! Perfect synchronization! These two ships are instantly communicating!"

But they aren't. They are just watching the same event. We call this Spurious Connectivity. It creates "ghost connections" that clutter our maps and make them useless for surgery.

The Skeptic's Tool: Phase Lag Index (PLI)

To banish the ghosts, we use the Phase Lag Index (PLI). The logic is brilliant: Electricity spreads instantly, but true brain communication takes time. It takes milliseconds for a signal to travel down an axon and jump a synapse.

Therefore, the PLI acts like a skeptical bouncer. It looks at two signals and says: "If you arrived at the exact same time (zero lag), I don't trust you. You're just an echo. I only count the signals where one clearly leads and the other follows."
$PLI = | \langle sign(sin(\Delta\phi(t))) \rangle |$

Zero Lag (Volume Conduction): The math ignores it.

Consistent Lag (True Synaptic Flow): The math counts it.

The Trade-off: Precision vs. Jitters

The PLI is conservative. Sometimes, it's too conservative. It throws out some real synchronization (sometimes brain areas do sync perfectly via the Thalamus). It can also be "jumpy" or high-variance.

To smooth this out, many of us are switching to Imaginary PLV (iPLV). Instead of a harsh "yes/no" switch, it uses the imaginary component of the cross-spectrum to gently filter out the zero-lag ghosts while keeping the data smooth.
$iPLV = | Im(N1n=1 \Sigma Nei\Delta\phi(n)) |$

The Result: The Small-World Collapse

Once we use these tools to clean the data, we can draw a true map of the epileptic brain.

A healthy brain is a "Small World"—a Goldilocks zone where neighborhoods chat locally, but information can travel across the brain quickly. It is flexible.

The pre-ictal epileptic brain loses this flexibility. It becomes a rigid lattice. It becomes "sticky." The path length increases, making it hard for the brain to process information, and the local clusters tighten until the network reaches a tipping point.

The Bottom Line

Seizures are not random. They are a failure of network dynamics.

The Paradox taught us that the brain disconnects globally to seize locally.

PLI/iPLV taught us to ignore the "ghosts" created by the skull to see the true synaptic conversation.

Only by combining these insights can we move from observing epilepsy to predicting it.

The Whispering Revolutionary: Functional Hubs and the Epileptic Coup

To truly understand the epileptic brain, we have to burn the old maps.

For a century, we treated the brain like a geography textbook: Here lies the land of Memory; there lies the province of Vision. But if you sit with a neuro-engineer watching live EEG data, the geography dissolves. The brain isn't a map of static islands; it is a bustling, 24-hour stock exchange. It is a social network.

And in this network, just like in high school or global politics, popularity matters.

1. The Architecture of Influence

In the brain's social network, most neurons are quiet suburbanites—they only talk to their next-door neighbors. But a select few are Hubs. These are the super-connectors, the influencers, the nodes that hold the entire system together.

Subtopic 4.4 isn't just about anatomy; it is a detective story. It investigates how Temporal Lobe Epilepsy (TLE) is not a random electrical storm, but a calculated coup led by a hub gone rogue.

2. The Math of Clout: Nodal Strength (Si)

In standard neurology, we obsess over amplitude (voltage). We look for who is shouting the loudest. But in network neuroscience, we don't care about volume; we care about influence.

To measure influence, we use a metric called Nodal Strength (Si).

The "Influencer" Analogy

Imagine a crowded room:

High Amplitude: A drunk person shouting in the corner. They are loud, but ignored.

High Nodal Strength: The charismatic leader whispering a plan. They aren't loud, but everyone stops to listen. They are synchronized with the room.

The Formula

We calculate this using the Phase Locking Value (PLV). PLV is essentially a measure of "dancing to the beat." If Node A and Node B fire at the exact same rhythm, their PLV is 1. If they ignore each other, it's 0.

The Nodal Strength of a specific node i is the sum of all its successful relationships:
Si=j · =iΣPLVij

The Translation: Si tells us how many other parts of the brain are currently listening to this specific node. It measures functional "clout."

3. The "Rich Club": The VIP Lounge

The brain is an expensive machine to run (it burns 20% of your daily calories). To save energy, the brain uses a "Rich Club" architecture.

The Rich Club is a group of high-strength hubs (the VIPs) that are densely connected to each other. They form a high-speed superhighway. If you see a red Ferrari, it's identifying a visual signal (occipital lobe) and sending it to your decision center (frontal lobe). It doesn't take backroads; it takes the Rich Club highway.

The Epileptic Hijack Normally, this highway makes you smart. In epilepsy, it makes you vulnerable. If a seizure starts in a remote village (a local node), it might stay small. But if the seizure breaks into the VIP room—the Rich Club—it gains access to the superhighway. Instantly, the localized spark becomes a generalized forest fire.

4. The Hippocampal Paradox: From Ghost to God

This is the most fascinating and terrifying dynamic in Temporal Lobe Epilepsy. We call it the Isolation-to-Domination Paradox.

If you have hippocampal sclerosis (scarring), your hippocampus acts like a sleeper agent.

Phase 1: The Ghost (Inter-ictal State)

99% of the time, the scarred hippocampus is a broken, lonely node. Because of the cell death, it uncouples from the network.

Nodal Strength (Si): Very Low.

Status: Isolated.

Network View: On the map, it looks dark. It's a ghost town.

Phase 2: The Dictator (Pre-ictal State)

Seconds before a seizure, the ghost wakes up. The very node that was isolated suddenly begins to force its neighbors into lock-step synchronization.

The Shift: The PLV skyrockets.

Nodal Strength (Si): It climbs vertically, surpassing every other node.

Status: Super-Hub.

5. Engineering Control: The "Rank-Order" Solution

So, how do we stop a dictator?

If we are building a brain implant (like the RNS System) to zap the seizure before it starts, we can't just look at voltage. If the patient laughs, sneezes, or goes to a rock concert, voltage goes up everywhere. We don't want to shock a patient for laughing.

The Solution: Rank-Order Algorithms

We don't look at the absolute value of the noise; we look at the Relative Rank.

Continuous Monitoring: The device constantly calculates Si for all electrodes.

The Ranking: It asks, "Who is the most influential node right now?"

The Trigger:

Scenario A (Rock Concert): The whole brain is loud, but the hippocampus is still ranked #20. No Action.

Scenario B (Pre-Seizure): The room is quiet, but the hippocampus jumps from rank #20 to #5, then to #1. FIRE.

By targeting the rank rather than the volume, we catch the seizure not when it gets loud, but when the network topology shifts—when the crowd turns to listen to the wrong leader.

Summary Table: The Functional Shift

Feature	Healthy/Inter-ictal State	Pre-ictal/Seizure State
Hippocampal Role	The "Ghost" (Isolated)	The "Super-Hub" (Dominant)
Connectivity (Si)	Low (Si≈0)	Extremely High (Si→Max)
Network Topology	Diverse, small-world chatter	Hypersynchronized rigid order
Engineering Fix	Ignore low rank	Detect high rank & Stimulate

Decomposing the Signal: Fourier, Wavelet, and Spectral Analysis

5.1 The Prism and the Echo: DFT & Power Spectrum

When we stare at raw EEG data, we are looking at a locked diary. The voltage trace—that jagged, manic line scrolling across the monitor—is secretive. It is the aggregate shout of billions of neurons, a chaotic choir where everyone is singing a different song at the same time.

To the naked eye, a pre-seizure brain often looks identical to a healthy one. To find the warning signs, we cannot simply watch the wave rise and fall. We have to shatter it.

We need to stop looking at Time and start looking at Frequency. This is the philosophy of decomposition.

The Centrifuge of Signal Processing

Imagine you are handed a green smoothie. You taste it. It's sweet, grassy, perhaps a bit tart. But can you tell me exactly how many grams of spinach vs. how many grams of apple are in it? No. You only experience the blend.

Spectral analysis is the centrifuge. It spins that voltage smoothie until the ingredients separate. It allows us to look at a specific second of brain data and say:

> "Ah, this moment is 60% deep, slumbering Delta waves, and only 5% sharp, analytical Gamma waves."

In epilepsy, this shift in perspective is everything. It is the difference between seeing a storm cloud and knowing the barometric pressure is dropping before the first cloud even appears.

The Mathematical Engine: The DFT

The vehicle for this transformation is the Discrete Fourier Transform (DFT). While we use the Fast Fourier Transform (FFT) in our code for speed, the DFT is the soul of the operation.

Let's look at the equation, not as a chore, but as a machine with moving parts:
$Xk=n=0\Sigma N-1xne-i2\pi kn/N$

The "Correlation Machine"

When I teach this, I strip away the Greek letters and ask students to visualize a lock and key.

xn (The Reality): This is your raw brain signal. The messy reality recorded by the electrode.

e−i... (The Probe): This represents a perfect, rotating cycle—a pure tone at a specific speed (k).

The Sum (Σ): This is the correlation. We are effectively rubbing the "perfect tone" against the "messy brain signal" to see if they line up.

Think of it like this: Imagine you are standing in a noisy stadium trying to hear if your friend is whistling a specific tune. The DFT is a filter that blocks out everything in the universe except that one specific pitch.

If the brain is "whistling" that tune (frequency k), the math returns a huge number. Resonance.

If the brain is silent at that pitch, the math returns zero. Silence.

We do this sweep for every possible frequency, building a complete fingerprint of the brain's current state.

Power Spectral Density (PSD): The Energy Audit

The DFT gives us a complex number (magnitude and phase). But when hunting for seizures, we care about force. We want to know: Where is the brain spending its metabolic cash?

We calculate the Power Spectral Density (PSD):
P(f)= | Xk | 2

By squaring the magnitude, we ignore the timing (phase) and focus purely on Power.

Why "Power" Equals "Danger"

In the language of neurons, Power is a proxy for Synchronization.

Low Power: Neurons are chatting casually, firing at different times. This is normal.

High Power: Neurons are chanting in unison. They are locking step.

When P(f) spikes, it means neural populations are being "recruited" into a massive, rhythmic hypersynchrony. This is the hallmark of a seizure.

The Phenomenon of Spectral Reddening

Here is the most poetic and chilling concept in seizure prediction: The Color of Noise.

If you plot the Power (Y-axis) against Frequency (X-axis) on a log-log scale, you don't get a flat line. You get a slope that drifts downward. This is the 1/f scaling law.

Pink Noise ($\alpha \approx 1$): This is a healthy brain. It sounds like a waterfall or rustling leaves. It is a perfect balance of low-frequency structure (memory) and high-frequency fizz (processing).

Red Noise (a>1.5): This is a brain in trouble.

The Pre-Ictal Shift

Minutes, sometimes hours before a seizure, the "color" of the brain signal shifts. The high-frequency "fizz" (gamma activity) dies out. The complex, multitasking ripples of the brain vanish. In their place, low-frequency, sluggish waves begin to swell.

The slope tilts. The signal "Reddens."

The Insight: This isn't just a change in numbers; it is a collapse of complexity. The brain is losing its ability to process information. It is becoming stupid, slow, and rhythmic.

Critical Slowing Down: The Physics of Vulnerability

Why does the spectrum redden? To understand this, we have to leave neuroscience and look at physics. We look at Critical Slowing Down.

Imagine a marble sitting at the bottom of a bowl.

The Deep Bowl (Healthy): If you flick the marble (a perturbation), it instantly snaps back to the center. The system is resilient. Fast recovery = High frequencies.

The Flat Plate (Pre-Ictal): As a seizure approaches, the "bowl" flattens out. The forces keeping the brain stable are weakening.

Now, if you flick the marble, it doesn't snap back. It wanders. It lazily drifts. It takes a long time to return to equilibrium.

The Memory of the System

This "laziness" manifests mathematically as Spectral Reddening. The brain has developed a "long memory." It cannot shake off disturbances.

Healthy Brain: Forgets the past quickly, ready for new input.

Pre-Seizure Brain: Holds onto the past. A small spark that should have been extinguished lingers, grows, and eventually ignites the fire.

Practical Implementation: The Spectrogram

We cannot analyze an hour of data at once. The brain changes too fast. We need to watch the movie frame by frame.

We use the Short-Time Fourier Transform (STFT):

Slice: We chop the signal into 1-second windows.

Taper: We smooth the edges (like fading in and out) to avoid mathematical errors.

Compute: We run the DFT on that single second.

Stack: We paste these slices side-by-side.

This creates the Spectrogram—a heatmap of energy over time. It allows us to watch the "Reddening" happen in real-time, seeing the warm colors of high energy drift from the top (high freq) to the bottom (low freq) as the seizure builds.

Summary: The Spectral Fingerprint

Feature	Healthy / Inter-Ictal	Pre-Ictal (Danger Zone)	The Human Meaning
Tone Color	Pink Noise (≈1/f)	Red/Brown Noise (>1/f1.5)	The signal is losing its "crispness."
Dominant Frequency	Balanced Mix	Low Frequencies (Delta/Theta)	The brain is sluggish and "chanting."
Resilience	High (Fast recovery)	Low (Critical Slowing Down)	The brain is "sticky"—it can't shake off sparks.
Energy	Low & Scattered	High & Concentrated	The neurons are marching in lockstep.

Part 1: The Blur of the Long Exposure

Why the Old Tools Failed Us

Imagine you are trying to photograph a hummingbird in flight. If you leave your camera shutter open for ten seconds (the "Long Exposure"), all you will get is a blurry streak of color. You know the bird was there, but you can't see its wings beat. You can't see the mechanics of flight.

For decades, the Discrete Fourier Transform (DFT) was our long-exposure camera. It is a brilliant tool for stationary signals—things that hum constantly, like a refrigerator. But the brain is not a refrigerator.

When a seizure approaches, the brain does not hum; it shrieks. It produces a "chirp"—a signal that accelerates in pitch and intensity rapidly.

The Trap: If we use the DFT on a 10-second window containing a 1-second seizure chirp, the math "smears" that 1 second of chaos across the full 10 seconds.

The Result: We see a 30Hz signal in the data, but we have no idea when it happened. In neurosurgery, "somewhere in the last ten seconds" isn't a diagnosis; it's a guess.

Part 2: The Microscope of Time (Wavelets)

Catching the "Ictal Chirp"

To fix the blur, we stopped using infinite sine waves and started using Wavelets.

Think of a sine wave as a continuous tone that never ends. Now, think of a Wavelet as a single heartbeat on an ECG monitor. It rises, peaks, and vanishes. Because it is finite, we can slide it along the timeline to see exactly when things change.

We use the Continuous Wavelet Transform (CWT). This is the mathematical equivalent of a high-speed camera that can also zoom in and out.

The Engine Under the Hood

The math here is poetic. We take our signal x(t) and probe it with a "Mother Wavelet" ψ.
$C(a,b)= \int -\infty \infty x(t) a 1 \psi*(at-b)dt$

Let's humanize these variables:

ψ (The Template): We usually use the Morlet Wavelet. Why? Because nature repeats itself. The Morlet wavelet looks almost exactly like the electrical spike of a firing neuron. We are using the brain's own language to listen to it.

b (The Time Slider): We slide the wavelet along the timeline. Did the spike happen now? How about now?

a (The Zoom Lens):

Large a: We stretch the wavelet out. We are looking for slow, rolling ocean waves (Delta rhythms).

Small a: We squash the wavelet down. We are looking for the buzzing of a bee (Gamma rhythms).

The Breakthrough: The output isn't a spectrum; it's a Scalogram. It allows us to see the seizure not as a smear, but as a rising diagonal line—the "chirp"—showing us exactly where the electrical storm began.

The Invisible Enemy: High-Frequency Oscillations (HFOs)

With Wavelets, we found something lurking in the dark: HFOs. For years, we filtered out everything above 70Hz, thinking it was muscle noise. We were wrong. We were filtering out the "smoke" before the fire.

Using CWT, we now hunt for Fast Ripples (250–500 Hz).

Normal Ripples: Soft bursts associated with memory. The sound of a working brain.

Fast Ripples: The buzzing of a "short circuit." These are clusters of neurons firing so fast they have lost control.

Clinical Reality: If you remove the brain tissue generating the big spikes, the patient might still have seizures. If you remove the tissue generating the Fast Ripples, you are often removing the root cause.

Part 3: The Geometry of Chaos (Graph Fourier Transform)

From "When" to "Where"

Wavelets solved the Time problem. But the brain is not a single wire; it is a massive, tangled city of connections. A seizure is a traffic jam that spreads. To understand it, we need a map of the city.

This is the Graph Fourier Transform (GFT).

We stop treating electrodes as isolated channels. We treat the brain as a Graph $G=(V,E)$, where electrodes are nodes and white matter tracts are the highways connecting them.

The Topology of a Scream

In classical signal processing, we analyze frequencies over time. In GFT, we analyze frequencies over structure.

We build the Graph Laplacian (L), which defines the "road network":
$L=D-A$

Where D is how connected a node is, and A is who it is connected to.

When we apply Fourier analysis to this graph (x^=UTx), we aren't measuring speed (Hz); we are measuring Smoothness.

The Dinner Party Analogy

To understand Graph Frequency, imagine a dinner party:

Low Graph Frequency (Consensus): Everyone at the table is nodding in agreement. If Person A is happy, their neighbor Person B is also happy. The "signal" changes smoothly across the table.

In the Brain: This is the healthy state (or the generalized seizure). The voltage changes gradually across connected regions.

High Graph Frequency (Discord): Person A is screaming, but Person B (sitting right next to them) is whispering. The difference between neighbors is extreme.

In the Brain: This is the Focal Onset.

The Seizure Story in Three Acts

By watching the GFT, we can see the narrative arc of a seizure before the patient even twitches.

Act I: The Peace (Interictal) The brain is dominated by Low Graph Frequencies. The network is cooperative.

Act II: The Rebellion (The Pre-Ictal Spike) Suddenly, a High Graph Frequency spike appears.

What happened? One node (the seizure focus) has gone rogue. It is firing violently, but its neighbors are trying to suppress it (inhibitory surround). The "voltage difference" between the rogue node and its neighbors is massive. This is the "Discord."

The Opportunity: This is the moment to strike. The enemy is isolated.

Act III: The Collapse (Generalization) The neighbors give up. They stop suppressing the rogue node and join it. The "Discord" vanishes, replaced by a terrifying Low Graph Frequency hypersynchrony. The whole choir is now screaming the same note.

The Silent Watchman: Inside the Logic of the Eratio

1. The Heartbeat of the Machine

Imagine a tiny titanium device, no larger than a matchbox, nestled inside the skull. It is a miracle of modern engineering, but it suffers from a very human problem: exhaustion.

Every time this device "thinks"—every time it runs a complex algorithm to analyze the brain's electrical storm—it burns energy. If it thinks too hard, too often, the battery dies. For the patient, a dead battery doesn't mean finding a charger; it means another neurosurgery, another incision, another recovery.

This creates a paradox. To be safe, the device needs to watch everything. To survive, it needs to sleep.

Enter the Energy Ratio Index (Eratio). It is the device's subconscious. It is a low-power reflex that allows the heavy-duty processor to sleep, waking it only when the whispers of the brain turn into a scream.

2. The Mathematics of "Calm" vs. "Storm"

We tend to think of seizures as chaos, but mathematically, they are often a brutal form of order—a synchronization where neurons stop doing their individual jobs and start chanting in unison.

To detect this without draining the battery, we don't look for shapes or complex patterns. We look at Energy Balance.

Think of a bustling coffee shop.

The Background: A low hum of conversation, clinking cups, and music. This is the brain's "Alpha" rhythm (idling).

The Event: Suddenly, a fire alarm goes off. The background hum vanishes, replaced by a singular, piercing tone. This is the "Epileptogenic" rhythm.

The Eratio is simply a comparison of the Alarm volume to the Coffee Shop volume.

$$Eratio=\Sigma\, Pbackground\, \Sigma\, Pepileptogenic$$

In Peace: The denominator (Background) is heavy. The ratio is tiny (<1.0). The device sleeps.

In War: The denominator collapses. The numerator (The Storm) spikes. The ratio explodes (>5.0). The device wakes up.

The Engineering Insight: We aren't looking for the seizure itself yet. We are looking for the imbalance that heralds its arrival.

3. Two Brains in One Box: The Sentinel and The Professor

To make this work, the implant actually possesses a split personality. This architecture is the secret to its longevity.

The Sentinel (The Reflex)

This is a tiny, primitive circuit. It consumes almost no power (microwatts). It is "dumb" in the sense that it can't learn or reason. It does one thing only: it watches the Eratio balance scale. It never sleeps. It is the guard standing at the gate, watching the horizon for dust.

The Professor (The Brain)

This is the powerful CPU. It runs Deep Learning models; it decides when to shock; it records data. But it is energy-hungry. Consequently, it spends 99% of its life in a deep coma.

The Interaction: The Sentinel watches the electrical waves. As long as the Eratio stays low, It lets the Professor sleep. But the moment the ratio crosses the "Red Line" (the threshold), the Sentinel kicks the Professor awake.

Sentinel: "Wake up! The energy balance just shifted 300%."

Professor (waking up in milliseconds): "Okay, let me analyze the signal... Yes, that's a seizure. Initiating therapy."

4. The "Red Line": The 3-Sigma Rule

How does the Sentinel know when to panic? We use the 3-Sigma Rule.

We analyze the patient's normal day—sleeping, eating, laughing. We find their average ratio (μ) and how much it naturally wiggles (standard deviation, σ).

We set the tripwire at:
$\text{Threshold} = \mu + 3\sigma$

Statistically, this means we are 99.7% sure that whatever is happening right now is not normal. It is the mathematical equivalent of saying, "This isn't just a weird noise; this is a gunshot."

5. Stories from the Edge: Clinical Reality

The math looks clean on paper, but inside a human being, it is a dramatic tug-of-war.

The "Slow Roll" (Mesial Temporal Lobe)

The Patient: A young man whose seizures start with a sense of déjà vu.

The Biology: His hippocampus begins a slow, rhythmic "pumping" in the Theta band (4–8 Hz).

The Sentinel's View: The "Background" Alpha hum fades. The slow "Theta" wave rises. The scale tips.

The Result: The Sentinel sees the ratio climb from 0.5 to 2.0. It triggers the wake-up. The Professor confirms it and stimulates. The patient feels the déjà vu evaporate instantly. He never loses consciousness.

The "Gamma Burst" (Cortical Dysplasia)

The Patient: A teenage girl with a miswired patch of motor cortex.

The Biology: A "Ripple"—a high-frequency buzz (High-Gamma) that acts like an electrical short circuit.

The Sentinel's View: Violent speed. The ratio jumps from 0.1 to 8.0 in the blink of an eye.

The Challenge: High-frequency noise can look like muscle movement (chewing). The Sentinel wakes the Professor, but the Professor must double-check: "Is this the brain, or is she just eating an apple?"

6. The Engineer's Burden

Designing the Eratio is an exercise in ethical geometry.

If we make the Sentinel too sensitive (low threshold), it wakes the Professor for every sneeze or stumble. The battery dies in two years. The patient undergoes risky surgery too soon.

If we make the Sentinel too strict (high threshold) to save the battery, it might ignore a subtle seizure. The device sleeps while the patient convulses.

The Eratio is not just an algorithm. It is a compromise between the finite limits of technology and the infinite complexity of the human brain. It is a silent pact we make with the patient: We will watch over you, but we will tread lightly, so that this guardian lasts as long as you need it.

The Fingerprint of Chaos: Lyapunov Exponents and Entropy

The Beautiful Storm: Why Your Brain Needs Chaos to Survive

We grow up believing that health is stability. We want a heartbeat steady as a metronome; we want a life that runs like clockwork. But if you look deep into the mathematics of the human brain, you find a terrifying truth: Clockwork is dangerous.

A healthy human mind is not a calm pond; it is a roiling ocean. It is a "Strange Attractor"—a mathematical storm that never repeats itself, constantly shifting, adapting, and reacting.

Conversely, an epileptic seizure is not chaos. It is the exact opposite. It is the imposition of a rigid, totalitarian order. It is the moment the ocean freezes solid.

To understand how we diagnose this difference, we have to look at the "Fingerprint of Chaos"—a number known as the Largest Lyapunov Exponent.

1. Mapping the Mind: The Phase Space

Before we do the math, imagine where the math lives. It lives in a conceptual arena called Phase Space.

Think of your brain's state as a single firefly moving through a dark room.

The Trajectory: The path the firefly flies.

The Attractor: The shape the firefly tends to stay inside.

In this room, there are three destinies for our firefly:

The Black Hole (Fixed Point): The firefly spirals into the center and stops moving. In the brain, this is coma or brain death. The lights go out.

The Nascar Track (Limit Cycle): The firefly gets stuck in a perfect loop. Round and round, exactly the same, forever. This is the seizure.

The Butterfly (Strange Attractor): The firefly zips around wildly. It never crosses its own path, but it stays within the room, tracing a beautiful, complex, non-repeating shape. This is you. This is consciousness.

2. The Mathematics of Separation: λ1

How do we distinguish the healthy "Butterfly" from the seizing "Track"? We measure how fast two moments separate from each other.

Imagine two thoughts that are almost identical.

In a seizure (Order): The two thoughts stay locked together, marching in step.

In a healthy brain (Chaos): The two thoughts diverge. One leads to a memory of breakfast, the other to a worry about an email. They drift apart rapidly.

The speed of this drift is the Lyapunov Exponent (λ1).

The Formula of " The Drift"

We model the distance d between two trajectories over time t as:

$d(t)=Ce\lambda1t$

To find the "fingerprint" ($\lambda1$), we ask: If I wait long enough, how fast does the gap widen?
$\lambda1=t\rightarrow\infty\lim d(0)\rightarrow0\lim t1\ln d(0)d(t)$

$\lambda1$ is the exponent. It tells us if the system is exploding (chaos) or collapsing (order).

ln (Natural Log) helps us decode the exponential growth.

3. The Spectrum of Control: Reading the Fingerprint

The value of $\lambda1$ is like a thermometer for the brain's flexibility.

$\lambda 1<0$: The Sinking Ship (Convergence)

If the number is negative, the trajectories are crashing into each other. The system is damping down.

The Vibe: A heavy blanket thrown over a drum kit.

The State: Deep anesthesia or coma. The brain is too stable to think.

$\lambda 1=0$: The Broken Record (The Limit Cycle)

The trajectories neither grow nor shrink. They are locked in a permanent orbit.

The Vibe: A marching band where everyone plays the exact same note at the exact same time.

The State: The Seizure. The neurons have stopped processing the outside world. They are only listening to their own internal echo. This is "hypersynchrony." The complexity of the mind collapses into a simple, repeating loop.

$\lambda_1 > 0$: The Jazz Improvisation (Chaos)

The trajectories push apart exponentially.

The Vibe: A jazz band. It's unpredictable, reactive, and complex. A small change (a trumpet note) shifts the whole mood (The Butterfly Effect).

The State: Health. A positive exponent means your brain is ready to pivot. If a tiger jumps out, you don't want to be stuck in a loop; you want to be able to switch states instantly. Chaos grants you the agility to survive.

4. The Pre-Ictal Drift: The Silence Before the Scream

The holy grail of epilepsy research is prediction. We want to catch the seizure before the shaking starts. The Lyapunov Exponent gives us a window into the future.

We look for a phenomenon called Dynamical Entrainment.

The Analogy of the Audience: Imagine a crowded theater before the show starts.

Healthy State (High λ_1): The roar of conversation. Everyone is saying something different. It is loud, chaotic, and information-rich.

Pre-Ictal (Dropping λ1): Slowly, a rhythmic clapping starts in the back row. People stop talking to listen. The "roar" dies down. The chaos fades.

Ictal/Seizure ($\lambda 1 \approx 0$): The entire audience is clapping in perfect unison. The conversation is dead. The complexity is gone.

When we monitor a patient's brain, we look for that drop in the exponent. We look for the moment the brain stops improvising and starts chanting.

5. Seeing the Unseen: Shadow Puppetry

How do we calculate this from a simple EEG wire on the scalp? We use a bit of mathematical magic called Takens' Theorem (Time Delay Embedding).

An EEG is a 2D flat line, but the brain is a multi-dimensional object. Takens' Theorem allows us to take that flat line and "unfold" it back into a 3D shape, like popping up an origami figure.

We take the voltage at this moment.

We take the voltage from a millisecond ago.

We take the voltage from two milliseconds ago.

By plotting these against each other, we reveal the "Shadow of the Attractor." We can see the shape of the chaos, even if we can't measure every neuron.

6. Entropy: The Volume of Information

Finally, we must look at Entropy. In information theory, entropy measures "surprise."

High Entropy (Health): The brain signal is full of surprises. This means it is carrying a lot of information (sights, sounds, thoughts).

Low Entropy (Seizure): The signal is totally predictable. A loop carries zero new information.

A seizure is an information blackout. The brain is shouting at the top of its lungs, but it isn't saying a single word.

Conclusion: The Kick

Understanding the "Fingerprint of Chaos" is changing how we treat epilepsy. We are moving away from just drugging the brain into submission.

Future devices, like the NeuroPace RNS, act like a conductor for that jazz band. By monitoring the Lyapunov Exponent in real-time, the device can sense when the "improvisation" is dying and the "chanting" is starting.

Just as the exponent drops, the device delivers a tiny electrical shock. This isn't to suppress the brain—it's to perturb it. It's a nudge. It kicks the record player so the needle skips out of the loop.

It forces the brain back into the beautiful, necessary storm of chaos.

The Symphony of Chaos: Why Your Brain Needs to Be Wild

Unlocking Subtopics 6.2 and 6.3

Introduction: The Lie of "Order"

There is a deeply held misconception that health equals order. We assume that a healthy heart beats like a metronome and a healthy brain is organized like a filing cabinet.

But when I first looked at the raw data of a healthy human brain, I didn't see a filing cabinet. I saw a riot.

The EEG of a healthy mind looks like static. It is jagged, rough, and seemingly random. For decades, neurologists dismissed this as "noise." But through the lens of non-linear physics, we learned the humbling truth: That noise is the sound of freedom.

A healthy brain is in a state of high-dimensional chaos. It is poised on a knife-edge, ready to react to a whisper, a shadow, or a sudden memory. It is infinitely flexible.

The terrifying paradox of epilepsy is that a seizure is not a descent into chaos. It is a collapse into rigid, totalitarian order. It is the moment the brain stops improvising and starts marching.

Subtopic 6.2: The Collapse (The Physics of the Soul)

If the healthy brain is a crowded cocktail party where everyone is having a unique, vibrant conversation, a seizure is the moment everyone stops talking and begins chanting the same word in unison.

To detect this, we look for the Loss of Complexity. We measure this using the Largest Lyapunov Exponent (LLE), denoted as $\lambda 1$.

The Divergence of Thought

The LLE measures the "Butterfly Effect"—how quickly two similar states drift apart.

The Wild State (Healthy): $\lambda 1 \approx 13$ bits/s. Information diverges rapidly. The system is exploring, reacting, feeling.

The Locked State (Pre-Ictal): $\lambda 1$ drops to ≈ 8 bits/s. The system is becoming sticky. Thoughts are trapped in a loop.

This drop is called Entrainment. It is the mathematical signature of neurons losing their individuality. They are being sucked into a "black hole" of synchronization—the Seizure Attractor.

Seeing the Ghost: Takens' Theorem

Here lies our biggest problem. The brain is a hyper-complex, 3D (or higher) monster. But our electrode is a simple wire giving us a 1D flat line of voltage.

How do you see a 3D monster through a 1D keyhole?

We use a beautiful piece of mathematics called Takens' Theorem. It operates on the principle of "Shadows and Memory."

Imagine watching the shadow of a dancer on a wall. You can't see the dancer, only the 2D shape. But, if you watch how the shadow moves over time, you can mentally reconstruct the 3D spin of the dancer.

We do this with data. We take the voltage now, and the voltage from a few milliseconds ago, and plot them against each other to "unfold" the hidden shape.

$Xn=[x(n),x(n+\tau),\ldots,x(n+(m-1)\tau)]$

We are essentially using the memory of the signal to reconstruct its geometry. But we must choose the right Embedding Dimension (m).

The Folded Map Analogy: If you try to draw a complex knot on a flat sheet of paper (m=2), the lines cross and it looks like a mess. You need to lift the lines up into the air (m=3 or higher) to see the true structure of the knot.

If we don't give the math enough dimensions ($m \geqslant 2D2+1$), the seizure's structure remains hidden in the knot.

Subtopic 6.3: The Engineer's Compromise (Survival Mode)

Subtopic 6.2 is the romanticism of Physics. Subtopic 6.3 is the brutal reality of Engineering.

In a lab with a supercomputer, calculating the LLE ($\lambda 1$) is easy. But we aren't in a lab. We are building a neurostimulator—a chip smaller than a postage stamp—implanted inside a human skull.

The Constraints:

Power: We run on a battery that needs to last years.

Heat: If the chip works too hard calculating complex math, it heats up. You cannot cook the brain tissue you are trying to save.

Calculating the true LLE requires heavy floating-point math (decimals, logs, divisions). It burns too much power. We needed a shortcut. We needed a way to measure "chaos" using simple arithmetic.

Enter Entropy: The Art of Surprise

We swapped the heavy physics of LLE for the lighter statistics of Sample Entropy (SampEn).

Think of the brain signal as a book.

The Seizing Brain: Reads like "The cat sat. The cat sat. The cat sat." (Low Entropy, Highly Predictable).

The Healthy Brain: Reads like Shakespeare. (High Entropy, Full of Surprises).

The formula looks like this:
$\text{SampEn}(m,r,N)=-\ln BA$

It's a matching game:

B: How many times does a specific pattern (like "1-2-1") appear?

A: How many times does that pattern continue in the same way (e.g., "1-2-1-3")?

If $A \approx B$, the brain is repeating itself. A seizure is coming.

Why We Abandoned ApEn (Approximate Entropy)

We used to use a metric called ApEn, but it had a fatal flaw: Ego. ApEn counted a vector as matching itself. It asked, "Do I look like me?" The answer is always yes. This bias skewed our data, especially on the short, bursty signals of an implant.

SampEn is honest. It removes the self-match. It demands real recurrence, not just a reflection in the mirror.

The "Chaos Meter" on a Chip

To save the patient, we strip the math down to its bones. We use FPGAs (Field-Programmable Gate Arrays). These aren't general-purpose computers; they are hardware circuits wired for one specific kill-shot.

We ditch the decimal points. We use integer arithmetic (1, 2, 3...). It is rough, it is jagged, but it is lightning fast and runs ice-cold.

When the FPGA sees the SampEn ratio drop—when the "Shakespeare" turns into "The Cat Sat"—it triggers the stimulation. It shocks the brain back into chaos. It restores the noise.

Summary

The transition from Subtopic 6.2 to 6.3 is the story of modern neurology.

6.2 teaches us that the brain is a high-dimensional, chaotic artist, and a seizure is the death of creativity (Entrainment).

6.3 teaches us that to save that artist, we must be pragmatic engineers. We cannot calculate the perfect shape of the storm (LLE) inside the skull, so we measure the predictability of the wind (SampEn) using simple tools.

We use the math of chaos to keep the brain wild.

The Brain is a Jazz Club, Not a Soldier's March

If you want to save a brain from a seizure, you first have to unlearn everything you know about "control."

We are taught that health is stability. We want our bridges rigid, our internet consistent, and our trains on time. But if you apply that logic to the human brain, you miss the point entirely.

A healthy brain is not a calm lake; it is a riot.

Imagine a dimly lit jazz club. The saxophone is doing one thing, the drums are doing another, and the piano is off on a wild tangent. To an outsider, it sounds messy. But to the musicians, it is a state of High-Dimensional Chaos. It is flexible. If the drummer changes tempo, the saxophonist adapts instantly. This is your brain on a good day.

Now, imagine a seizure.

A seizure is not the music getting "messy." A seizure is when the jazz band suddenly stops playing, stands up, and begins marching in a rigid lockstep, playing the exact same single note, over and over, at deafening volume.

A seizure is not chaos. A seizure is the tyranny of order.

To predict and stop seizures, we don't look for the storm. We look for the silence that comes before it.

I. The Metric of Freedom: STLmax

We cannot just "look" at brainwaves and guess if they are jazzy or rigid. We need a speedometer for chaos. We need a number that tells us: How free is this brain right now?

This is the STLmax (Short-Term Maximum Lyapunov Exponent).

Let's strip away the heavy calculus. The STLmax measures divergence. It asks a simple question about the future: If two thoughts start at nearly the same place, how quickly do they drift apart?

The mathematical relationship looks like this:
$\delta Z(t) \approx e \lambda t$

Where λ (lambda) is the Lyapunov exponent.

High STLmax ($\lambda > 0$): The "Butterfly Effect" is active. The system is wild, creative, and adaptable. The brain is safe.

Low STLmax ($\lambda \approx 0$): The system is stuck. The leaves on the river aren't separating. The brain is becoming a machine. Danger.

The Insight: We use "Short-Term" (STL) because the brain changes its mind every few seconds. We need to catch the mood swing the moment it happens, not an hour later.

II. The Premonition: Dynamical Entrainment

Here is the breakthrough that changes everything. The brain doesn't just "snap" into a seizure. It slowly gets sucked into it.

We call this Dynamical Entrainment, but let's call it "The Dip."

Think of the seizure focus (the damaged part of the brain) as a charismatic but boring speaker at a party.

The Healthy State: The party is loud. 50 different conversations are happening. (High STLmax).

The Entrainment: The boring speaker starts talking. Slowly, the people near him stop their conversations to listen. The room gets quieter. The "chaos" drops.

The Gradient: This silence spreads. The "Dip" in STLmax appears in one specific spot (the focus) and tries to pull the rest of the brain into its boring rhythm.

The Seizure: The whole room is silent, listening to the one speaker. The party is over.

The Window of Opportunity: Crucially, we can see "The Dip" on the monitors 30 to 90 minutes before the seizure physically happens. The brain is screaming a warning: "I am losing my flexibility! I am becoming too ordered!"

III. The Villain: The Dynamical Focus

Not all brain tissue is guilty.

In this theory, we are hunting for the Dynamical Focus. This is the "Bad Neighborhood" in the brain.

When we place electrodes on a patient, we see a Spatial Gradient (a slope).

The Focus: Shows the lowest STLmax (most rigid).

The Neighbors: Show medium STLmax.

The Rest of the Brain: Shows high STLmax (healthy chaos).

The Focus is a bully. It has low entropy (low randomness) and it essentially forces the healthy, high-entropy neurons to march to its drumbeat. It recruits them into the conspiracy of order.

State	Healthy Brain	Pre-Seizure Brain
Analogy	A busy market	A regimented army
STLmax	High (Positive)	Dropping (The Dip)
Behavior	Independent, flexible	Synchronized, rigid
Prediction	Impossible to predict (Random)	Highly predictable (Deterministic)

IV. The Cure: Healing with Noise

This is where the science sounds like magic.

If the problem is "Too Much Order," the cure must be Disorder.

Traditional medicine tries to sedate the brain (calm it down). But if the brain is already becoming rigid and silent, sedation acts like a red light at a traffic jam—it just stops movement.

The STLmax control strategy suggests we need to act like a riot instigator.

The Protocol:

Watch: The computer monitors the STLmax in real-time.

Detect: It sees "The Dip." The bully is starting to preach.

Attack: The device delivers a burst of Chaotic Stimulation (electrical noise) directly to the focus.

We don't zap the brain to shut it up. We zap it to wake it up.

We inject "noise" to break the lockstep. We disrupt the synchronization. It's like throwing a handful of marbles onto the floor of that marching band. The soldiers stumble, the rhythm breaks, and they are forced to stop marching and start jazzing again.

The Paradox: We use chaos to stabilize the patient. We use noise to restore the melody.

Summary: From Reactive to Preemptive

For the patient, this shifts the paradigm from Fear to Freedom.

Current devices wait for the seizure to start, then try to put out the fire. The Spatiotemporal/STLmax approach sees the wood drying out an hour beforehand. It rains on the wood (injects chaos) so the fire never sparks.

We are not just treating a disease; we are restoring the beautiful, unpredictable, chaotic complexity that makes us human.

The Rhythm of Rebellion: Kuramoto Dynamics and Synchronization

The Mathematics of the Mob: When the Brain Starts Chanting

To understand the chaos of a seizure, we first have to unlearn a common misconception: we tend to think of seizures as "electrical storms," implying random, noisy violence.

But a seizure isn't noise. It is the opposite. It is hyper-order.

Imagine a bustling jazz club. The saxophone is improvising, the drummer is off-beat, the piano is exploring a new chord. It sounds chaotic, but it is rich, complex, and functional. This is your healthy brain.

Now, imagine that abruptly, every single musician stops playing their song and begins slamming a single note, in perfect unison, at maximum volume. Bang. Bang. Bang.

That is a seizure. It is the moment the complex democracy of the brain collapses into a totalitarian chant. To understand how this happens, we turn to the Kuramoto Model—the mathematical story of how individuals surrender to the mob.

Part 1: The Cast of Characters

The Kuramoto model treats the brain not as a computer, but as a collection of oscillators—things that cycle over and over again, like a pendulum, a firefly, or a neuron.

To solve the mystery of the mob, we have to meet the three distinct personalities vying for control inside your head.

1. The Runner: The Phase (θ_i)

"Where am I?" Imagine a runner on a circular track. The variable θ (theta) is simply where they are on that loop.

In the Brain: It represents the neuron's specific moment in its firing sequence. Is it resting? Is it charging up? Is it spiking?

2. The Ego: Natural Frequency (ω_i)

"I want to run at my own pace." Left to their own devices, every neuron has a preferred speed. This is ω (omega).

The Healthy Conflict: In a vibrant brain, you want disagreement. You want the visual cortex running at a different speed than the auditory cortex. Diversity of speed creates complexity of thought.

3. The Peer Pressure: Coupling Strength (K)

"Do what everyone else is doing." This is the villain and the hero of our story. K represents how much attention a neuron pays to its neighbors.

The Balance: If K is too low, the neurons ignore each other (coma/confusion). If K is too high, the neurons lock together (seizure).

Part 2: The Tug of War

The mathematical equation that governs this behavior is a literal tug-of-war. It calculates the "velocity" of a neuron—how fast it is moving around the track.
$\dot{\theta}i=\omega i+NKj=1 \sum N\sin(\theta j-\theta i)$

Let's translate this from math into human behavior.

The Drive for Independence (ωi): The first part of the equation says: "I am going to move at my own speed." If there were no connection to others, this is all that would matter.

The Social Pull ($NK\sum \sin(\ldots)$): The second part says: "But I am being pushed and pulled by the crowd."

If my neighbor is ahead of me, the math pulls me forward to catch up.

If my neighbor is behind me, the math drags me back to wait for them.

The Insight: Every millisecond, your neurons are fighting a battle between their Ego (ω) and the Peer Pressure (K). In a seizure, the peer pressure wins. The voice of the individual is drowned out by the shout of the group.

Part 3: The Watcher on the Wall

How do we know who is winning? We use a mathematical tool called the Order Parameter, denoted as $r(t)$. Think of this as the "Volume Knob" of the brain's synchronization.

$r(t)ei\psi(t)=N1j=1 \Sigma Nei\theta j(t)$

Don't let the exponents scare you. Visualizing it is simple:

The Healthy Whisper ($r \approx 0$): Imagine a crowd pointing arrows in random directions. If you average them all out, they cancel each other. The net result is zero. The brain is humming quietly, processing a million different thoughts.

The Seizure Scream ($r \approx 1$): Imagine the crowd suddenly turning and pointing their arrows at the exact same target. They add up. The "volume" hits maximum.

Part 4: The Tipping Point (The Millennium Bridge)

The scariest thing about the Kuramoto dynamics is that the change isn't gradual—it is a Phase Transition. It happens in the blink of an eye.

The most famous real-world example isn't in a brain, but on a bridge.

In 2000, the Millennium Bridge opened in London. As thousands of people walked across, the bridge began to sway slightly. To keep their balance, pedestrians unconsciously adjusted their steps to match the sway.

The Sway acted as the Coupling Strength (K).

The Steps synchronized.

The Result: The more they synchronized, the harder the bridge swayed. The harder it swayed, the more they synchronized.

Within minutes, a crowd of strangers locked into a terrifying, unified march. The bridge had a seizure. In epilepsy, the "sway" is the electric field. Once it gets strong enough, neurons have no choice but to march to the beat.

Part 5: The "Chimera" and The Fatigue

Modern computational neuroscience has found two fascinating wrinkles in this story that give us hope.

1. The Chimera State

For years, we thought the brain was either Sync (Seizure) or Async (Healthy). Recently, simulations revealed the Chimera State: a ghostly condition where half the brain is seizing, and the other half is normal. This perfectly models focal seizures. It is a "partial rebellion," where a rogue neighborhood starts a riot while the rest of the city goes about its business. Detecting these "fractures" in the network is the new frontier of prediction.

2. Why the Riot Stops (The Fatigue Hypothesis)

Why doesn't a seizure last forever? In our simulations, we view the "Natural Frequency" (ω) not as a constant, but as a battery.

The seizure starts.

Neurons fire rapidly, chanting in unison.

They get tired. They run out of metabolic energy.

Their "Ego" slows down. They can no longer keep up with the fast pace of the mob.

The synchronization breaks.

The rebellion fails because the rebels exhaust themselves.

Conclusion: The Beauty of Chaos

The Kuramoto model teaches us a profound philosophical lesson about our own biology. We usually crave order and structure in our lives. But inside our skulls, order is dangerous.

Health is a state of "metastability"—a delicate, dancing balance where we are synchronized enough to understand the world, but chaotic enough to remain individuals.

We need the noise. We need the jazz. Because when the noise stops and the chanting begins, the music is over.

The precarious Edge: Order, Chaos, and the Chimera

If you were to stand inside a living brain, it wouldn't sound like a well-oiled machine. It would sound like a crowded cocktail party. Thousands of voices—neurons—are chattering away, each with its own rhythm, its own distinct pitch. This clamor, this "noise," is what keeps us alive. It is the sound of possibility.

But the brain is constantly fighting a gravitational pull toward a darker state. It exists on a knife-edge. Lean too far into chaos, and thoughts scatter like dust. Lean too far into order, and the cocktail party stops. Everyone starts chanting in unison. The clamor becomes a roar. This is the seizure.

In the physics of the brain, we study this battle using the Kuramoto model, specifically focusing on the moment the battle is lost: the Phase Transition.

7.2 The Cliff Edge: Phase Transitions and the Cost of Perfection

We tend to think of disease as a gradual decline. But in nonlinear dynamics, the brain behaves less like a dimmer switch and more like water turning to ice. One moment it flows; the next, it is solid. This is the Phase Transition.

The governor of this transition is a parameter called Coupling Strength (K). Think of K as "peer pressure" between neurons. It is the force that encourages them to sync up.

There is a mathematical line in the sand, a specific threshold called Critical Coupling (K_c).

Safety Zone ($K<K_c$): The neurons listen to each other but keep their own rhythm. We are conscious.

The Danger Zone ($K>K_c$): The peer pressure becomes too strong. Individual rhythms collapse into a collective lock-step. We seize.

The Mathematics of Conformity

The formula for this tipping point reveals a profound biological truth:

$K_c=\pi g(0)2$

The term g(0) measures the uniformity of the neurons. A "tall" or high g(0) means the neurons are all virtually identical—clones of one another.

The Insight: The formula tells us that if neurons are too similar (high g(0)), the threshold K_c drops to the floor. It takes almost nothing to push them into a seizure.

The Human Lesson: Health requires diversity. A resilient brain is a messy brain, full of neurons with different natural frequencies and quirks. When the brain becomes too homogenized, it loses its defense against the "mob mentality" of synchronization.

The Cruel Irony of Learning (The "Trojan Horse")

Here lies the tragedy of the human condition. The mechanism that makes us intelligent is the same one that pushes us toward the cliff edge.

We call it Hebbian Learning: "Neurons that fire together, wire together." When you learn to play the violin, your brain tightens the connections (K) between specific neurons to make the task easier. You are optimizing your neural pathways. You are increasing efficiency.

But to a physicist, "increasing efficiency" is just a polite way of saying "increasing Coupling Strength (K)." Epilepsy, in this light, is not always a failure of the brain. Often, it is a brain that has optimized itself too well. It has learned so efficiently, strengthened its bridges so robustly, that it has eliminated the safety buffer of chaos. The "Kindling" phenomenon is simply the brain drifting, day by day, closer to Kc, until the silence of the pre-ictal state gives way to the storm.

7.3 The Chimera State: The Paradox of partial Seizure

For a long time, we thought the brain had two modes: On or Off. Sync or Async. Awake or Seizing.

Then, the math showed us something impossible. We call it the Chimera State. Named after the beast from Greek mythology—part lion, part goat, part snake—this state is a hybrid monster.

In a Chimera state, the brain is split:

The Coherent Domain: A knot of neurons locked in a high-voltage seizure.

The Incoherent Domain: The rest of the brain, buzzing along happily, completely unaware of the disaster next door.

The Invisible Fire

This is the mathematical portrait of a Focal Seizure. Imagine a patient sitting across from you. Their left hand is trembling rhythmically (the Coherent Domain), yet they are speaking to you calmly, maintaining eye contact, perhaps even solving a riddle (the Incoherent Domain).

The danger of the Chimera is that it is mathematically camouflaged. If we use standard tools to measure the Global Order Parameter (the average synchrony of the whole brain), the math lies to us.

The seizure implies $r \approx 1$.

The healthy part implies $r \approx 0$.

The average is a low, unassuming number.

To a standard algorithm, the brain looks normal. But locally, a fire is burning. The healthy neurons act as an "entropy sink," absorbing the disorder and hiding the seizure from the global view.

The Researcher's Reality: A Moment of Dread

From the lab notes of a computational neuroscientist:

"There is a specific feeling of dread that comes from watching a Chimera state emerge in a simulation. We were running a model based on a patient's connectivity data. For hours, the screen showed the comforting 'fuzz' of a healthy brain—like the static of a detuned radio.

Then, we tweaked the coupling just slightly, simulating sleep deprivation.

It didn't explode. It curdled.

A pocket of nodes in the temporal lobe suddenly snapped into a rhythmic, high-amplitude lock-step. It was hypnotic and terrifying. But the rest of the brain? It just kept humming. The frontal lobe didn't care. The parietal lobe didn't notice.

I looked at the global output numbers. They barely moved. If I had been a monitor in a hospital room relying on that average, I would have told the nurse the patient was sleeping peacefully. Meanwhile, inside the model, the patient was screaming.

It changed how I see the brain. We aren't searching for global storms anymore. We are hunting for pockets of rogue order hiding inside the chaos. We have to stop looking at the whole ocean and start looking at the waves."

The Next Step: Local Detection

To find a Chimera, we must abandon the global view. We must break the brain down into its communities and listen to the local whispers. We calculate the Local Order Parameter:

rlocal(k)=Nk1j∈CkΣeiθj

We scan the brain neighborhood by neighborhood, hunting for the high r values hiding in the shadows of the low global average.

The Jazz Club Paradox: Defining the Enemy

Close your eyes and imagine a busy jazz club. The drummer is doing one thing, the saxophonist another, the patrons are chatting in small groups. It sounds chaotic, but it is information-rich. This is your brain when you are thinking, feeling, and being human.

Now, imagine that suddenly, every single person in that club—musicians, waiters, patrons—stops what they are doing and slams their hand on the table at the exact same millisecond. Bang. Bang. Bang.

That is a seizure.

We tend to fear chaos, but in neuroscience, order is the killer. A seizure is pathological perfection. It is Hypersynchrony, where the diversity of thought collapses into a totalitarian rhythm. To cure it, we don't need to restore order; we need to restore the beautiful mess of individuality.

The Old Way: The Firehose

Historically, when the brain started "banging on the table," our medical response (Standard Deep Brain Stimulation) was to scream through a megaphone. We blasted the brain with high-frequency electricity. It worked, but it was exhausting. It drowned out the seizure, but it also drowned out the subtle music of the mind.

The New Way: The Whisper

Demand-Controlled Desynchronization is different. It is a sniper, not a shotgun. It waits in the shadows, watching the math. It only acts when necessary, and it uses the neuron's own momentum against it.

The Mathematics of Peer Pressure (The Kuramoto Model)

To stop the mob, we must quantify it. We use the Kuramoto Model, which essentially writes the "Equation of Peer Pressure" for neurons.

$$\dot{\theta}_i = \omega_i + Kr\sin(\psi - \theta_i) + I_{stim}(t)$$

Let's translate this equation into the characters of our story:

The Individual (θ_i): This is the single neuron. It has its own phase (where it is in its cycle).

The Personality (ω_i): This is the neuron's natural rhythm. Left alone, it wants to dance to this beat.

The Mob Leader (r and ψ):

r is the Order Parameter. It measures how strong the mob is (0 = Jazz Club, 1 = North Korean Military Parade).

ψ is the Mean Field Phase. This is the rhythm the mob is chanting.

The Peer Pressure (K): The coupling strength. This is the force pulling the individual to join the mob.

The Mechanism of the Seizure: When the term $Krsin(\psi-\theta i)$ becomes too strong, the individual neuron surrenders. It stops following its own personality (ωi) and locks into the mob (ψ). The seizure begins.

The Strategy: The Judo Throw

We cannot easily change the neuron's personality (ω) or the brain's connectivity (K). So, we introduce a new character: The Intervenor (Istim).

The goal of Demand-Controlled Desynchronization is to minimize the order parameter (r). We want to drive the derivative negative ($\dot{r}<0$). We want to crash the system.

1. Timing is Everything (The Phase Response Curve)

Imagine a child on a swing.

If you push them at the bottom of the arc, you make them go faster (adding energy).

If you push them at the top of the arc, you barely add speed, but you change their timing.

This is the Phase Response Curve (PRC). We don't want to add energy (that might make the seizure worse). We want to change the timing. The device monitors the Mean Field Phase (ψ) and waits for the precise millisecond where the neurons are "at the top of the swing."

Then, it delivers a micro-nudge.

2. Coordinated Reset (CR): Breaking the Phalanx

Standard stimulation hits everyone at once. But if you push a marching army all at once, they just march in a new direction. You haven't broken the formation.

Coordinated Reset (CR) is deviously smart. It splits the electrode into four distinct contacts (A, B, C, D).

> Nudge Contact A: Group A stumbles.
>
> Wait 5ms... Nudge Contact B: Group B stumbles.
>
> Wait 5ms... Nudge Contact C: Group C stumbles.

By staggering the hits, we force the neurons out of alignment. We aren't silencing them; we are confusing them. We turn the marching army back into a scattered crowd. The r value crashes to zero. The seizure evaporates.

The "Cure": Unlearning the Habit

This is the most "human" part of the mathematics.

The brain is plastic. It follows the rule: "Neurons that fire together, wire together." When a brain has epilepsy, it has learned to seize. The pathways for synchronization are paved highways.

Standard stimulation just puts up a roadblock. But Coordinated Reset actually tears up the pavement.

By constantly forcing the neurons to fire out of sync (Desynchronization), we trigger Spike-Timing-Dependent Plasticity (STDP) in reverse:

> "Neurons that fire out of sync, lose their link."

Over time, the brain unlearns the seizure. The coupling strength (K) between these pathological neurons weakens naturally. Even if you turn the device off, the patient often remains seizure-free for long periods. This is the Anti-Kindling Effect.

Summary: The Shift in Perspective

Feature	The Old Way (Standard DBS)	The New Way (Demand-Controlled)
Philosophy	Suppression (Hold the door shut)	Re-education (Teach the door to close)
Metaphor	The Megaphone	The Whisper
Energy Use	Continuous (High Battery Drain)	On-Demand (High Efficiency)
Mechanism	Overpowering the Neurons	Exploiting the Phase Response Curve
Long Term	Dependence	Potential Remission (Plasticity)

The Warning Whisper: Critical Slowing Down and Autocorrelation

The Art of Forgetting: Mathematics, Resilience, and the Warning Whisper

In the neurology ward, fear creates its own distinct silence. For a patient living with epilepsy, the seizure itself—violent and chaotic—is often less terrifying than the peace that precedes it. The peace is a lie. It is an ambush. This uncertainty hangs like a heavy curtain, turning everyday joys—holding a newborn, boiling water for tea, walking down concrete stairs—into potential tragedies.

For a long time, we treated the brain like a static machine and seizures like lightning strikes: bad luck, sudden, emerging from the void. But the brain is not a machine; it is a choir. And before the choir descends into screaming chaos, it doesn't just snap. It hesitates. It drags.

The brain whispers before it screams. We just had to learn the language of the whisper. It turns out, the grammar of that whisper is written in Calculus.

The Physics of "Letting Go"

To understand how a seizure starts, we have to rethink what it means to be "healthy." We often think of health as strength, rigid and unyielding. But in dynamical systems—whether it's the stock market, the climate, or your temporal lobe—health is actually amnesia.

Imagine a marble sitting at the bottom of a deep, round bowl.

The Healthy State: You flick the marble (a stressor, a missed night of sleep, a flashing light). The marble shoots up the side, but gravity immediately snaps it back to the bottom. The system "forgets" the flick instantly. It resets. It is resilient.

The Pre-Seizure State: Now, imagine the bowl begins to melt. It becomes a flat platter. You flick the marble. It doesn't roll back. It wanders. It drifts sluggishly. It "remembers" the push and refuses to settle.

This sluggishness is a phenomenon physicists call Critical Slowing Down (CSD). When a system is about to crash, it loses its gravity. It loses the ability to pull itself back to center.

The Mathematics of the Echo

We cannot physically touch this "bowl" inside the skull. We have to measure the shape of the bowl using the shadows it casts on an EEG monitor. To do this, we use a beautiful, terrifyingly simple piece of mathematics called the Lag-1 Autocorrelation (AR-1).

We model the brain's electrical narrative with this equation:

$$xt+1=a1xt+\sigma\epsilon t$$

Let's humanize this equation. It is a story about the Past, the Future, and the Grip.

The Now (xt) and The Next (xt+1): This is the timeline. Where is the brain's voltage now, and where will it be a millisecond from now?

The Noise ($\sigma \epsilon t$): This is the chaos of being alive. A car honking, a neuron misfiring, a sudden thought. This is the "flick" of the marble.

The Grip ($a1$): This is the ghost in the machine. This coefficient measures how much the Current Moment is clutching onto the Previous Moment.

The Danger of a Perfect Memory

Here lies the counter-intuitive truth: A healthy brain shouldn't remember its own electrical noise.

In a healthy brain, $a1$ is low (close to 0). A perturbation hits, and the brain sheds it. It moves on. It is flexible.

In a pre-seizure brain, $a1$ climbs toward 1. The brain becomes sticky. It becomes rigid.

When $a1 \to 1$, the system stops correcting itself. Think of driving a car with broken suspension.

Healthy ($a1=0.2$): You hit a bump. Thud. Gone. The ride smooths out.

Critical ($a1=0.99$): You hit a bump. The car bounces. While it's bouncing, you hit another bump. The bounces stack on top of each other. The car begins to oscillate wildly. You lose control.

As the correlation coefficient ($\rho 1$) rises, the brain is essentially trapping itself in an echo chamber. The "restoring force"—the biological gravity that keeps us sane—vanishes.

$$\rho 1=\sigma 2E[(xt-\mu)(xt+1-\mu)]$$

When this value creeps up, the brain is signaling that it is too tired to fight the entropy. It is ready to collapse.

The Algorithm in the Wild

In my research, I hunt for this creeping number. But the real world is messier than a textbook.

We use a "sliding window" technique. Imagine looking at a frantic painting through a tiny cardboard tube, moving it inch by inch across the canvas. We analyze 60 seconds of brain data, calculate the "stickiness," slide the window forward, and calculate again.

We found that hours before a seizure, the trend line often shifts. Patient A might hover at a safe 0.5. Then, slowly, quietly, it climbs. 0.6... 0.75... 0.8. The brain is screaming, "I can't let go. I can't process this noise."

The False Alarm Dilemma There is a catch. Deep sleep also looks like Critical Slowing Down. When you dream, your brain waves slow; they become correlated. If we aren't careful, an alarm would go off every time a patient took a nap. To solve this, we must build context into the math. We don't just look for "high numbers." We look for "high numbers when you should be awake." We look for the anomaly.

Reclaiming the Stove

Why does this abstract algebra matter?

It matters because of the young woman who is afraid to cook dinner. She fears the seizure that strikes while the gas is on.

If we can translate

$x_{t+1} = a_1 x_t$

into a wrist-worn device, we change her life.

Scenario: She wants to cook. She checks her status. The algorithm sees her a_1 is low. The "bowl" is deep. She is safe. She cooks.

Scenario: Two hours later, the device buzzes. The algorithm detects the "stickiness" rising. The bowl is flattening. The Whisper is audible. She turns off the stove. She lies down on the carpet. The seizure comes, but she is safe.

The Final Variable

Ultimately, this research suggests something profound about existence.

Resilience—whether in a stock market, an ecosystem, or a human mind—is not about holding on tight. It is about the ability to let go. It is the ability to absorb the shock of the world and return to center.

By listening for the moment the brain loses this flexibility, by tracking the rise of a_1, we are doing more than predicting seizures. We are giving people back the ability to trust their own timeline. We are turning a catastrophe into a calendar event, and in doing so, handing the controls back to the pilot.

The Tremor Before the Quake: Listening to the Brain's Whispers

For decades, treating epilepsy felt like chasing ghosts. We were like meteorologists who only started paying attention once the tornado was already tearing the roof off. By the time a seizure hits—the "storm"—the neurological damage is already in motion. It is violent, chaotic, and loud.

But nature rarely screams without whispering first.

There is a moment before the chaos—a silent, mathematical shift in the atmosphere—known as Critical Slowing Down. It is the sound of the brain losing its grip, not yet falling, but struggling to stand. Our research has moved from watching the storm to measuring the pressure in the air.

Here is how we are decoding the language of a brain on the brink.

Part 1: The Exhausted Dancer (Variance and Autocorrelation)

To understand what happens before a seizure, forget the complex diagrams for a moment. Instead, imagine a tightrope walker.

In a healthy brain, the rope is taut. The walker is rested. If a gust of wind (biological noise) hits them, they correct their balance instantly. The movement is sharp, fast, and barely noticeable. They possess resilience.

In a pre-seizure brain, the rope goes slack. The walker is exhausted. This loss of tension—the flattening of the "potential well"—leads to two distinct warning signs that we can see in the data.

The First Whisper: The Brain Gets "Sticky" (Autocorrelation)

In statistics, we call this Lag-1 Autocorrelation (a1), but let's call it System Memory.

A healthy brain lives in the now. It processes a signal and moves on immediately. It is agile. But as a seizure approaches, the brain gets "sticky." It becomes nostalgic. It holds onto the past state for too long.

Think of it like driving a sports car versus a heavy truck:

The Sports Car (Healthy): You tap the brakes, the car responds, and you're back to speed instantly. The "memory" of the brake tap vanishes.

The Heavy Truck (Critical): You tap the brakes, and the momentum drags. The vehicle is sluggish. The impact of that one action lingers for seconds, affecting everything that follows.

When we look at brain waves, we see this sluggishness. The jagged, energetic static of a healthy brain turns into slow, rolling waves. The brain has lost its snap. The mathematical value of a1 creeps toward 1, telling us: "I am tired. I cannot let go of this disturbance."

The Second Whisper: The Wandering Path (Variance)

This creates a paradox. The brain is reacting slower (high autocorrelation), but it is also swaying wider (high variance).

Return to our tightrope walker on the slack rope. Because the rope is loose, they can't find their center.

Healthy: The walker stays within an inch of the center line.

Critical: The walker swings two feet to the left, then two feet to the right.

The "restoring force"—gravity, or the brain's natural inhibition—is gone. The background noise of the brain (ϵt) stops being a hum and becomes a force that pushes the brain around.

We express this terrifying relationship with this equation: $Var(x)=1-a12\sigma2$

Look at the bottom part: ($1-a12$). As the "stickiness" ($a1$) grows and gets closer to 1, the bottom of that fraction gets closer to zero. In mathematics, as you divide by zero, the result shoots toward infinity.

Translation: As the brain's resilience hits zero, the chaos becomes infinite. The tightrope walker falls.

Part 2: The Gentle Nudge (Active Probing)

The methods above are passive. They require us to sit quietly and watch the tightrope walker sway. But what if the wind isn't blowing? What if the brain is too quiet to show us its instability?

We cannot afford to wait for luck. We need to ask the brain a question.

We call this Active Probing, but you can think of it as Sonar for the Soul.

The Radar Approach

Instead of listening to the brain's natural noise, we use an implanted device to send a tiny, imperceptible electrical pulse—a "ping"—into the cortex.

We aren't trying to shock the brain; we are just tapping it on the shoulder to see how fast it turns around. We measure the Decay Rate, modeled by lambda (λ):

$$x(t) \propto e^{\lambda t}$$

The Healthy Response (High Negative λ): You tap the brain, and it absorbs the energy instantly. It's like throwing a pebble into thick mud—it lands with a thud and stops. The system is stable.

The Critical Response (λ near 0): You tap the brain, and it rings like a bell. The energy echoes. It lingers.

Measuring the Distance to the Cliff

This is the ultimate game-changer. Passive listening tells us "The weather looks bad." Active probing tells us, "You are exactly 50 meters from the cliff edge."

By measuring how long that "ping" echoes, we can mathematically calculate the distance to Bifurcation—the point of no return where a seizure begins. It transforms epilepsy management from a guessing game into an engineering problem. We don't have to guess if the patient is unstable; we can measure it, calibrated and precise, regardless of whether the patient is sleeping, running, or reading.

The Future: From Reaction to Conversation

We are moving toward a world where neuro-implants are not just firefighters putting out blazes; they are guardians.

They will constantly query the brain: "Are you okay? Are you resilient?" And if the brain whispers back, "I am tired, I am slowing down," the device can intervene—adjusting stimulation to tighten the rope and deepen the bowl—hours before the first tremor of a seizure is ever felt.

Subtopic 8.4: The Flickering Phenomenon – Anatomy of a Neural Storm

Introduction: The Ghost in the Machine

Imagine standing on a suspension bridge during a high wind. The bridge is solid, engineered to hold massive weight. But every now and then, a gust hits it at just the right angle, and you feel a shudder—a vibration that lasts a second too long. It stabilizes, but for that brief moment, the structure wasn't just existing; it was negotiating with gravity.

We have traditionally viewed seizures as sudden, lightning-strike events—a binary switch that flips from ON to OFF. But the neuroscience of Subtopic 8.4 suggests otherwise. The brain does not simply collapse; it flickers. Like a fluorescent light bulb struggling to stay on before it finally burns out, the neural networks oscillate between stability and chaos.

This transitional phase offers us the most promising window for prediction we have ever found. It allows us to move from asking "Will a seizure happen?" to observing "The seizure is already trying to happen."

Part I: The Lived Experience – "I Feel It Coming"

To understand the science, we must first ground it in the reality of the patient. In neurology, we talk about "prodromes" and "auras," but these clinical terms often fail to capture the visceral reality of a brain in a state of bistability (flickering).

Interviews with patients often reveal a hauntingly consistent narrative. It isn't pain. It is a profound sense of fragility.

> "It feels like my thoughts are skipping a beat. I can carry on a conversation, but the background noise in my head gets louder. It's like a radio tuner that is drifting slightly off-station. It flickers back to clear sound, then static, then clear again. And I know, if the static stays for more than a few seconds, I'm gone."

This subjective experience aligns perfectly with the objective physics. That "skipping a beat" is the neural network jumping between a normal firing pattern and a seizure-like pattern, but not yet committing to the seizure. It is testing the waters.

Part II: The Physics of the Flicker (The Landscape)

To understand how a seizure happens, we have to stop thinking of the brain as a computer and start thinking of it as a dynamical landscape.

Picture a landscape with two valleys (or "basins of attraction"):

- Valley A (The Green Valley): This is the healthy state. The "ball" (your brain's current state) rolls around in the bottom of this valley. It is safe here. If you push the ball up the hill a little bit (stress, a flashing light), gravity rolls it back down to the bottom. This is resilience.

Valley B (The Dark Valley): This is the seizure state. If the ball falls into this valley, it gets stuck in a loop of high-amplitude, synchronous firing.

In a healthy brain, the hill between Valley A and Valley B is a mountain. It is impossible to cross. But in an epileptic brain, the landscape shifts. The mountain erodes into a small hill.

The Flickering Phenomenon occurs when the ball is sitting on the very top of that ridge, being kicked back and forth by the noise of biology.

Kick left: You feel normal.

Kick right: You feel "off," or the EEG shows a spike.

Kick left: Normal again.

Part III: The Warning Signs – Variance and Autocorrelation

How do we detect this invisible flickering before the seizure actually happens? We look for two specific mathematical "ghosts" that appear in the data: High Variance and Critical Slowing Down.

1. High Variance (The Wild Swings)

Imagine a heart rate monitor. A healthy heart rate varies, but within a predictable, tight range. As a system approaches a tipping point, it loses its "tightness." The control mechanisms loosen.

In the brain, this manifests as neuronal firing rates that swing wildly. Instead of a gentle hum, the EEG shows bursts of loud activity followed by silence. The brain is swinging the steering wheel wildly just to keep the car on the road.

2. High Autocorrelation (The Memory of Chaos)

This is the subtler, deadlier sign. This is often called Critical Slowing Down.

Healthy State: If you poke a healthy brain (e.g., a flash of light), it reacts and immediately forgets it. It returns to baseline instantly.

Pre-Seizure State: As the transition nears, the brain becomes "sticky." If a neuron misfires, that misfire hangs around in the system. The state at Time T becomes highly predictive of the state at Time T+1.

The Metaphor: Think of a mattress. A firm, new mattress (Healthy) bounces back instantly when you stand up. An old, worn-out memory foam mattress (Pre-Seizure) leaves a dent that takes a long time to recover. When the brain loses its elasticity, the seizure is near.

Part IV: The Power Law and The "Fat Tail"

This brings us to the most sophisticated method of prediction. If you measure the duration of these "flickers"—how long the brain spends in the micro-seizure state before popping back to normal—you might expect a standard Bell Curve. You would expect most flickers to be very short, with almost no long ones.

But nature loves a Power Law.

In the pre-seizure state, the distribution of flicker durations shifts. It develops a "Fat Tail".

Normal Distribution: The probability of a long flicker is effectively zero.

Power Law Distribution: The probability of a long flicker drops off much more slowly. Extreme events become far more likely.

Why this matters: When the math shifts from a Bell Curve to a Power Law, it proves that the "energy barrier" keeping the brain safe has collapsed. The brain is no longer visiting the seizure state by accident; it is being magnetically pulled toward it.

Part V: Summary of the Phenomenon

To consolidate this into a clear framework, let's look at the progression from health to storm:

Stage	The Physics	The Feeling (Subjective)	The Data (Objective)
1. Baseline	Deep valley of health. High resilience.	"I feel fine."	Low variance. Fast recovery from stimulation.
2. The Drift	The valley gets shallower. Resilience drops.	"I feel tired, stressed, a bit 'off'."	Autocorrelation starts to rise (Critical Slowing Down).
3. The Flicker	Bistability. Jumping between states.	"My thoughts are stuttering. Déjà vu."	Bursts of High Variance. Flickers follow a Power Law.
4. Transition	The barrier collapses.	Loss of awareness.	Seizure onset. High amplitude synchrony.

Conclusion: The Future of Prediction

The "Flickering Phenomenon" teaches us to look for the wobble before the explosion.

Modern neuro-implants (like the RNS System) are moving toward detecting these specific statistical shifts. They aren't just counting spikes; they are calculating the variance of the noise.

If we can detect the flicker—the moment the brain starts to "stutter"—we can intervene. A precisely timed electrical pulse delivered during a "flicker" can act like a hand steadying the canoe. It pushes the brain back into the healthy valley before the permanent transition occurs.

The Control Knobs: Network Controllability and Gramians

9.1 Core Formula: Controllability Gramian (Wc)

The Physics of Changing Your Mind

For centuries, neuroscience has been cartography. We drew maps of the brain, naming the ridges of the cortex and the valleys of the hippocampus. But a map is static. It tells you where the cities are, not how much gas it takes to drive between them.

If the structural connectome (the white matter wiring) is the road map, Network Control Theory (NCT) represents the traffic dynamics. It answers the fundamental human question: What is the metabolic cost of moving from a state of deep depression to a state of joy?

The mathematical heart of this answer is the Controllability Gramian (Wc).

Part I: The Philosophy of Steering

To understand the Gramian, we must abandon the metaphor of the brain as a desktop computer. A computer is rigid; you press 'A', and 'A' appears.

The brain is more like a turbulent ocean. Neural activity is the water—constantly shifting, flowing, and crashing. You—the conscious observer, or the clinician—are the captain of a ship on this ocean. You want to steer. But you cannot steer arbitrarily. You are constrained by two things:

The Currents (A): The structural connectivity (white matter tracts) that dictates natural flow.

The Rudder (B): The input matrix, determining where we can actually inject energy (sensory input or stimulation).

The Controllability Gramian is neither the ship nor the rudder. It is the chart of the currents. It mathematically defines the "Energy Landscape" of your mind. It tells us which mental states are "downstream" (easy to reach) and which are "uphill" (energetically expensive).

Without the Gramian, we are blind captains. We might try to steer a patient out of a tremor, only to find we are pushing against an immovable wall of physics. With the Gramian, we can calculate the cost of the journey before we ever set sail.

Part II: Deconstructing the "Time Machine" Equation

Let's strip the fear away from the calculus. This equation is a narrative of how energy ripples through time.

The brain is a Linear Time-Invariant (LTI) system defined as:
$\dot{x}=Ax+Bu$

$\dot{x}$: How your brain state changes this millisecond.

A: The roads (white matter).

B: The entry points (stimulation).

The Controllability Gramian W_c over a time horizon T is:

$$W_c(T)=\int_0^T e^{A\tau}BB^Te^{A^T\tau}\,d\tau$$

Let's break this dense narrative down:

1. The Ripple Effect ($e^{A\tau}$)

The term $e^{A\tau}$ is the matrix exponential. In plain English, this is propagation. If you pluck a guitar string (perturb a neuron), the sound waves ripple out, bouncing off the wood and interfering with each other. This term captures that ripple. It calculates how an input at "time zero" travels through the complex web of white matter to affect the rest of the brain at time τ.

2. The Port of Entry (BB^T)

The matrix B defines where the energy enters. The term BB^T acts as a filter. It acknowledges that we cannot control the brain from everywhere. We are limited to specific ports of entry (eyes, ears, or a TMS coil). This term restricts the math to reality.

3. The History ($\int_0^T \ldots d\tau$)

Integration is just fancy addition. We are summing up every possible ripple effect from the moment the stimulus starts until time T. The Gramian is a cumulative history of possibility.

The Result: W_c is a matrix that summarizes "reachability."

Large W_c: The system is open. You can steer it anywhere.

Small/Singular W_c: The system is caged. No matter how hard you push, certain states are mathematically impossible to reach.

Part III: The Energy Landscape (Valleys and Peaks)

This is the most vital framework for understanding the "lived experience" of mental health. Imagine your brain's state space not as numbers, but as a physical terrain.

Valleys (Basins of Attraction): These are comfortable states. The brain naturally rolls here. (e.g., Deep sleep, the Default Mode Network, or a chronic depressive episode).

Peaks: These are high-energy, unstable states. (e.g., Panic, complex cognitive switching, intense focus).

The Eigenvalues of the Gramian (λ) map this terrain.

Large Eigenvalues (λ_{large}): These align with the valleys. Moving the brain this way is like floating downstream. It costs almost zero energy.

Small Eigenvalues (λ_{small}): These correspond to steep cliffs. Moving the brain in these directions requires massive energy input to fight the structural connectivity.

The minimum energy (E_{min}) required to reach a specific target state (x_f) is:
$E_{min}=x_f^T W_c^{-1} x_f$

Note the Inversion (W_c^{-1}): If the Gramian is small (small eigenvalues), the inverse becomes huge. This explains why breaking a habit feels physically exhausting. You are trying to climb a mathematical cliff.

Part IV: Two Flavors of Control

In applying this theory, we've found that "control" isn't a monolith. Your brain uses two distinct strategies, analogous to two types of athletes.

1. Average Controllability: The Marathon Runner

Calculated by: Trace of the Gramian (sum of eigenvalues).

The Vibe: Stability, endurance, maintenance.

The Location: The Default Mode Network (DMN) and structural hubs.

The Function: These nodes act as Peacekeepers. They steer the brain into "easy," low-energy states. When you are meditating or daydreaming, you are relying on high average controllability. They keep the system running smoothly in the valleys.

2. Modal Controllability: The Sprinter

Calculated by: Eigenvectors of the Gramian (focusing on small eigenvalues).

The Vibe: Disruption, agility, switching.

The Location: Frontoparietal Control Network (FPN) and executive areas.

The Function: These nodes are Circuit Breakers. They are structurally positioned to drive the brain into difficult, high-energy states. When you hear a loud bang and switch from "sleep" to "fight," you are engaging Modal Controllability. You are forcing the brain over a mountain pass.

Part V: Clinical Reality and Lived Experience

How does this linear algebra translate to the human condition?

Case Study A: The "Stuck" Brain (Depression)

In major depression, the energy landscape warps. The "valley" of sadness deepens.

The Math: We often see alterations in Average Controllability in the limbic system.

The Reality: The patient feels "heavy." This isn't a metaphor; it's a control-theoretic reality. The energy required (E_{min}) to reach a state of "motivation" exceeds the brain's metabolic budget. They are mathematically trapped in a gravity well.

Case Study B: The Flattened Landscape (Psychedelics)

Studies on psilocybin via NCT show a phenomenon called Landscape Flattening.

The Math: The drug perturbs the functional coupling, effectively making the eigenvalues of W_c more uniform. The difference between "easy" and "hard" directions shrinks.

The Reality: Boundaries dissolve. Thoughts that usually feel "impossible" (small eigenvalues) become accessible. The rigid mountains of the ego are leveled into a rolling plain.

Case Study C: The Black Hole (Epilepsy)

A seizure is a state of such high gravity (stability) that once the brain drifts near it, it inevitably falls in.

The Math: In Temporal Lobe Epilepsy, the brain loses the "Modal" ability to switch away from the seizure focus.

The Fix: Surgeons can use the Gramian to identify which nodes have control authority over the seizure focus, targeting them for ablation to "raise the walls" of that valley.

Part VI: The Future of Medicine

We currently treat the brain chemically (flooding the whole engine with oil) or electrically (zapping a general area). The Gramian offers a path to Prescribed Dynamics.

Imagine a future where we scan your connectome and compute your personal Gramian. We see that your anxiety exists because the energy cost to move from Amygdala-High to Prefrontal-High is 20% higher than average due to a specific weak tract.

Instead of generic pills, we prescribe a precise pattern of stimulation (u(t)) designed to lower that specific energy barrier. We aren't there yet, but the Gramian is the map that will get us there.

Summary Table

Concept	Symbol	The Analogy	The Lived Experience
Structural Matrix	A	The Roads	Your physical brain wiring.

Input Matrix B		The Doorway	Where stimuli enter (senses/TMS).
The Gramian	Wc	The Map	The catalog of what is possible.
Large Eigenvalues	λmax	Downstream	Habits, flow, ease.
Small Eigenvalues	λmin	Uphill	Focus, breaking habits, change.
Average Control	Tr(Wc)	The Marathoner	Staying stable (Peacekeeping).
Modal Control	ϕi	The Sprinter	Switching tasks (Revolutionary).

The Cartography of Consciousness: Navigating Brain States

When we view the brain through Network Control Theory (NCT), we stop looking at anatomy books and start looking at a topographical map. We are no longer seeing "tissue"; we are seeing a dynamic, shifting terrain—a vast energy landscape.

Imagine your brain is a mountain range. Every state of being—from deep sleep to solving a calculus problem to suffering a seizure—is a specific coordinate on this map.

To move from one coordinate to another requires Control Energy. This isn't just the glucose your brain burns; it is the specific computational effort required to steer billions of neurons from one pattern to another.

In my work with patient connectomes, I have come to view epilepsy not as a random storm, but as a navigational hazard. The brain gets trapped in a "gravity well"—a deep valley it cannot climb out of. To save the patient, we have to become the navigators.

Part 1: The Engines of Navigation

To move across this landscape, we have two very different types of engines. In the math of control theory, these are Average and Modal controllability. In plain English, they are the Conformists and the Rebels.

1. Average Controllability (The Conformists / The Hubs)

These are the loud, popular nodes of the brain—the "Rich Clubs" like the Precuneus or Anterior Cingulate Cortex. They are connected to everyone.

The Math: Mathematically, this is defined by the trace of the controllability Gramian: Average Controllability $\propto \mathrm{Trace}(W_c)$.

The Vibe: When you stimulate a Hub, it acts like a loudspeaker. The signal washes over the whole brain instantly. They are excellent at maintaining the status quo and keeping the brain synchronized.

The Trap: You might think, "To stop a seizure, hit the biggest hub!" But this is dangerous. Seizures are states of hypersynchrony. Since Hubs are designed to synchronize the brain, stimulating them can actually push the patient deeper into the seizure valley.

2. Modal Controllability (The Rebels / The Whisperers)

These are the quiet nodes sitting on the periphery of the network—areas in the frontal pole or lateral temporal cortex. They aren't famous, but they hold a secret power.

The Math: This metric comes from the eigenvectors of the adjacency matrix. It is inversely related to eigenvalues: Modal Controllability $\approx \sum_{j=1}^{N}(1-|\lambda_j|^2)\phi_{ij}^2$.

The Vibe: These nodes are specialists. They are weak at maintaining the status quo, but they are incredibly powerful at breaking it. They are the "levers" that can push the brain into difficult, desynchronized states.

The Savior: Because a seizure is a "trap" of synchronization, we need a Rebel to break it. Stimulating these peripheral nodes kicks the brain out of the valley and forces it into the complex, "difficult" state of normal consciousness.

Feature	Average Controllability (Hubs)	Modal Controllability (Peripheral)
Role	The Broadcaster	The Specialist
Location	Densely connected core	Sparsely connected edges
Superpower	synchronizing the group	Breaking the consensus
Epilepsy Use	Avoid (May worsen seizure)	Target (Aborts seizure)

Part 2: The Paradox of Energy

To understand why we target the "Rebels" (Modal nodes), you must understand the Energy Paradox of the brain.

Visually, a seizure looks violent—wild spikes on an EEG. It looks like high energy. But from a control theory perspective, a seizure is a path of least resistance. It is a low-energy basin. It is the brain collapsing into a simple rhythm because it is "tired" of maintaining the complex, high-energy state of being awake.

The Reality: Consciousness is the hard work. The seizure is the collapse.

Therefore, our therapy shouldn't try to "calm" the brain (which stabilizes the collapse). We need to inject energy to push the brain back up the hill. We need to desynchronize it.

Part 3: Boundary Controllability (The Fire Doors)

While the previous section dealt with resetting the whole brain, Subtopic 9.3 deals with Containment.

Many patients suffer from Focal Epilepsy. The seizure starts in a specific spot (the focus) and then spreads like a wildfire. The danger isn't the spark; it's the spread.

Boundary Controllability is the science of finding the "Gatekeepers."

The Virtual Resection

Traditionally, if a surgeon wanted to stop the spread, they would physically cut the connections (corpus callosotomy). They would burn the bridge. But we can do better. We can use "Virtual Resection."

Map the Terrain: We view the brain as two rooms: Room A (The Fire/Focus) and Room B (The Healthy Brain).

Find the Door: We analyze the Gramian of the partitioned system to find the specific nodes that act as the bridge between A and B.

Lock the Door: Instead of cutting the tissue, we place an electrode on that boundary node. When the seizure starts, we stimulate that node to "clamp" it.

The result? The seizure burns itself out in the focus, but it cannot cross the bridge. The patient remains conscious, perhaps unaware that a seizure even occurred. We haven't extinguished the fire; we've just closed the fire door.

Part 4: The Rational Battle Plan

By synthesizing these concepts, we move from "blind stimulation" to Rational Network Control. We now have a tactical flowchart for next-generation neurostimulation:

Is the seizure contained?

Yes: Use Boundary Controllability. Target the gatekeepers. Clamp the edges. Keep the fire small.

Has the seizure escaped and generalized?

Yes: Use Modal Controllability. Ignore the hubs. Target the peripheral "Rebels." Inject high energy to kick the brain out of the valley and restore the complex rhythm of consciousness.

This is the future of neurology: treating the brain not just as biology, but as a navigable landscape where we can choose the destination.

Subtopic 9.4: The Breathing Matrix and the Pre-Ictal Paradox

The Lie of the Static Map

If you open a standard neuroscience textbook, you will see diagrams of the brain that look like intricate subway maps. Node A connects to Node B. The lines are solid. The structure is permanent.

This is a beautiful, comforting lie.

In the reality of the operating room, staring at the raw data washing over the monitors, you learn the truth: The brain is not a sculpture; it is a swarm. The connectivity matrix—that mathematical roadmap we call A—is not etched in stone. It breathes. It fluctuates. It is a living, time-varying entity.

In control theory, we usually assume the roads stay put. But in an epileptic brain, the roads themselves are twisting, breaking, and reforming in milliseconds. This is the challenge of Time-Varying Controllability. We are trying to navigate a map that changes while we are driving on it.

The Paradox: When the Orchestra Freezes

Here is the phenomenon that keeps neuroengineers awake at night. It is the "Pre-Ictal Paradox," and it defies intuition.

As a seizure approaches (the pre-ictal phase), the brain stops its usual chaotic, healthy multitasking. Normally, your neurons are like a cocktail party—thousands of little localized conversations happening at once. But as the seizure looms, the room goes silent. The neurons begin to synchronize. They start chanting in unison.

This creates a bizarre trade-off in our ability to control the brain with a pacemaker:

1. The "Easy" Part: Average Controllability Spikes Imagine a regiment of soldiers marching in perfect lockstep. If you shove the whole group, the whole group moves. Because the brain has locked into this synchronized state, it is paradoxically easier to push the entire system around. The "average" energy needed to move the brain state drops.

2. The "Impossible" Part: Modal Controllability Crashes Here is the trap. While you can move the whole regiment, try getting just one soldier to break step and do a jumping jack. It's impossible. The peer pressure (synchrony) is too strong. This is Modal Controllability. The seizure "mode" is rigid. The stiffness of the system prevents us from isolating and targeting the specific bad pattern. We can push the brain, but we can't finesse it.

The Visual: Imagine a flat sheet of paper (the normal brain state). You can crumple it, fold it, move any part of it. Now imagine that paper collapsing into a tight, hard tube (the seizure state). You can roll the tube easily (Average Controllability), but you can no longer bend the paper (Modal Controllability).

The Mathematics of a Moving Target

To understand why this is an engineering nightmare, we have to look at the math. In classical engineering, we use a static equation:

$\dot{x}=Ax+Bu$

We assume A (the brain's map) is constant. But because the brain is plastic and reactive, we are actually fighting a Linear Time-Varying (LTV) system:

$\dot{x}(t)=A(t)x(t)+B(t)u(t)$

This small (t) changes everything. Our "fuel gauge"—the Controllability Gramian (Wc)—is no longer a static number we can look up. It becomes a dynamic history of the system's movement, an integral that shifts every millisecond:

$$W_c(t_0,t_1)=\int_{t_0}^{t_1}\Phi(t_1,\tau)B(\tau)B^T(\tau)\Phi^T(t_1,\tau)\,d\tau$$

Translated: Our ability to steer the brain depends not just on where we are, but on the exact path the brain took to get here. The window of opportunity is transient.

The Energy Landscape: The "Valley of the Seizure"

Why does the seizure become so hard to stop once it starts? I call this the Dimensionality Collapse.

The Plateau (Normal Life): When you are thinking, dreaming, or working, your brain exists in a high-dimensional space. It's wandering a vast, flat plateau. It takes very little energy to move from one thought to another.

The Valley (The Seizure): As synchrony rises, the neural trajectory falls off the plateau and slides into a deep, steep valley (an attractor).

The Energy Crisis: Once the brain is at the bottom of this valley, the walls are incredibly steep. To "lift" the brain out of the seizure state (to break the mode) requires an exponential amount of energy.

If we stimulate too late, the energy required to kick the brain out of the valley exceeds what our battery-powered implant can deliver without burning the tissue.

The Grand Challenge: Racing the Clock

This brings us to the human reality of the loop. We are designing algorithms that sit on a chip inside a skull, trying to predict the future.

Calculating the optimal control path requires solving complex matrix math (roughly O(N3) complexity) in real-time. But we can't fit a supercomputer in a patient's chest. We have a low-power battery and milliseconds to act.

The "Hacks" We Use to Survive:

The Snapshot: We pretend the brain stops moving for 1 second. We take a picture of A(t), solve the math for that static picture, and fire.

The Lookup Table: We memorize the "shape" of the pre-seizure valley. When the device sees the brain entering that specific canyon, it doesn't do math—it just fires "Plan B," which we pre-calculated on a laptop weeks ago.

Summary: The Closing Window

The Metric	The Shift	The Narrative Meaning
Synchrony	Increases	The crowd stops talking and starts chanting.
Avg. Controllability	Increases	The system becomes loose and drifty.
Modal Controllability	Decreases	The specific seizure pattern hardens like concrete.
Energy Cost	Spikes	The price of escape skyrockets.

The Lived Experience For the neuroengineer, the "Pre-Ictal" phase isn't just data. It's a countdown. When you review the logs, you see the system screaming. You see the spectral power shift, the matrix tighten, and the "Valley" form. You know the algorithm has perhaps 5 seconds to inject a pulse before the mathematics of the system renders it uncontrollable—before the lock-in is complete.

It is a high-stakes negotiation with chaos.

Seeing in the Dark: State Estimation and Kalman Filters

The Mathematical Whisperer: Decoding the Brain's Static

Part 1: Flying Blind in the Biological Storm

Close your eyes. Imagine you are piloting a plane through a hurricane at midnight. The windshield is painted black. The horizon is gone.

You have no visual on the mountains ahead. All you have is a dashboard of flickering, rusty dials. The altimeter sticks. The compass spins wildly every time lightning strikes.

This is the daily reality of a neural engineer.

We tend to think of brain surgery as the pinnacle of precision, but the electrical reality is messy. The brain is a universe of 86 billion neurons—a hidden state, $x(t)$, of infinite complexity. To listen to it, we lower clumsy microphones (electrodes) into the soup.

But these microphones don't give us the truth. They give us $y(t)$—a distorted echo. The signal is buried under the roar of muscle movements, the 60Hz hum of the wall outlets, and the mechanical shifting of the wire itself.

To treat a patient—to stop a tremor in Parkinson's or catch a seizure before it starts—we cannot rely on these lying dials. We need a co-pilot. We need a mathematical entity that can look at the chaos, remember the laws of physics, and whisper: "Ignore the lightning. We are actually here."

That co-pilot is the Kalman Filter.

Part 2: The Algorithm of Trust

At its heart, the Kalman Filter isn't just an equation; it is a philosophy of Trust Management.

It operates on a cycle of anxiety and relief. It constantly asks a profound question: Who do I trust more? My internal belief about how the world works, or the noisy evidence right in front of my eyes?

Let's trace the heartbeat of this algorithm as if it were a living, thinking engine.

Phase I: The Prediction (The "Gut Feeling")

Before the sensors even deliver data, the filter makes a bold prediction. It relies on "physics memory." If a brain wave was rising a millisecond ago, momentum says it should keep rising.

The mathematical intuition looks like this:

$$x_{k \mid k-1} = A x_{k-1 \mid k-1} + B u_{k-1}$$

The Translation:

x (The State): The filter says, "Based on the past, I bet the brain is here."

A (The Physics): The laws of motion. It knows that brain waves usually ripple, they don't teleport.

B (The Action): If we just zapped the brain with electricity (u), we expect a reaction. B maps the shock to the result.

But the filter is humble. It knows biology is messy. So, it calculates a Fog Index:

$P_{k|k-1} = A P_{k-1|k-1} A^T + Q$

P (The Anxiety): How scared are we? A high P means we are flying through thick fog.

Q (The Chaos Factor): This is the "Ghost in the Machine." It acknowledges that neurons misfire and chemicals fluctuate. Q tells the filter: "Expect the unexpected. The universe is random."

Phase II: The Update (The Reality Check)

Now, the sensor beeps. A measurement (y_k) arrives. It's ugly, jagged, and noisy. The filter must decide how much to listen to it.

Enter the Negotiator, also known as the Kalman Gain (K):
$K_k = P_{k|k-1} H^T (H P_{k|k-1} H^T + R)^{-1}$

Think of K as a slider bar between Arrogance and Naïveté.

R (Measurement Noise): This is the quality of our microphonc.

If R is high (Garbage Sensors): The Gain (K) drops to zero. The filter covers its ears, ignores the data, and trusts its own prediction.

If R is low (Precision Sensors): The Gain (K) rises. The filter admits, "I was wrong, the data is right," and corrects course.

Finally, the reconciliation happens:
$x_{k|k} = x_{k|k-1} + K_k (y_k - H x_{k|k-1})$

The term ($y_k - H x_{k|k-1}$) is the Innovation. It represents Surprise. It is the difference between what the filter expected and what it saw. The Kalman Gain takes that surprise, scales it, and uses it to update reality.

Part 3: Stories from the Neural Void

Why does this abstract math matter? Because for a patient in a hospital bed, these variables translate directly to quality of life.

Case A: The "Ghost" in the Wire (Parkinson’s Disease)

The Scenario: You have a Deep Brain Stimulation (DBS) implant. We want to zap the brain only when a "beta burst" (a rigidity signal) appears. The Problem: You are walking down the street. The cable in your neck wiggles. This creates a massive electrical spike that looks like a beta burst, but is actually just a loose wire artifact. Without Kalman: The device sees the spike, thinks "Parkinson's!", and zaps you unnecessarily. You might slur your speech or feel a tingle. With Kalman: The filter analyzes the spike against the matrix A (physics). It realizes: "This spike is moving too fast to be a brain wave. It breaks the laws of biology." The Gain (K) drops. The system ignores the cable noise. You keep walking, symptom-free, and the battery is saved.

Case B: The Blanking Period (Epilepsy)

The Scenario: A "smart" pacemaker for the brain detects a seizure and fires a counter-pulse to stop it. The Paradox: The moment the device fires, the loud electrical shout deafens its own sensors. For a few milliseconds, the system is totally blind (The Blanking Period). The Kalman Fix: This is the filter’s finest hour. Even though the sensors are dead (no y), the prediction step (Ax) keeps running. The filter flies on autopilot, estimating the brain's trajectory through the darkness. When the sensors wake up, the co-pilot is still on course, ready to resume control.

Part 4: The Art of the Tune

Textbooks teach you the formulas. Experience teaches you the Art.

A neural engineer spends their life "tuning" the matrices Q and R. It is a personality test for the machine.

The Paranoid Tuner (High Q): You tell the filter the brain is volatile. The estimate becomes jittery, chasing every shadow. Good for catching fast seizures, but exhausting.

The Stubborn Tuner (High R): You tell the filter the sensors are liars. The estimate becomes smooth, like a slow river. It looks nice, but it reacts too slowly to save a patient from a sudden attack.

In the most advanced systems, we use Adaptive Kalman Filters. This is where the math becomes biological. The filter realizes that the brain while sleeping is different from the brain while doing math. It rewrites its own matrices (A, Q, and R) in real-time. It evolves.

Conclusion

The Kalman Filter is often taught as linear algebra. It is not.

It is the bridge between the analog chaos of our biology and the digital precision of our machines. It allows us to reach into the dark, noisy void of the human mind and pull out a clear, actionable signal. It turns the static into a symphony, giving the patient back their control, their movement, and their life.

Whispers in the Dark: Mapping the Hidden Brain

Introduction: The Biological Ocean

We often make the mistake of thinking the brain is a computer. It isn't. A computer is a flat, logical grid of circuits, laid out where we can see them.

The human brain is more like a deep, biological ocean. It has surface waves, yes, but it also has trenches, caverns, and currents moving in the pitch black of the deep. For decades, we tried to understand epilepsy by floating rafts on the surface—placing electrodes on the outer cortex. We assumed that if we watched the waves on top, we'd know what the ocean was doing.

We were wrong.

Deep down, in the buried valleys of the hippocampus (memory) and the insula (emotion), storms can rage while the surface remains calm. By the time that storm breaches the surface, the patient is already lost to the seizure.

To fix this, we don't just need better sensors; we need better philosophy. We need the Kalman Filter.

Part I: Hunting the Phantom (The "Hidden" Seizure)

The Problem: The Room Behind the Door Imagine a locked room. Inside, a fight breaks out. Outside, you are pressing your ear against the heavy door. At first, you hear nothing. The fight (the seizure) is happening, but the door (the brain tissue) muffles the sound. You only realize there is a problem when the fighters crash into the door, busting it open.

In neurology, this is the "blind spot." A patient might feel a wash of fear or nausea—an aura—signaling a seizure in the deep insula. They know it's coming. But the surface electrodes? They read flat. They are deaf to the whisper; they are waiting for the shout.

The Solution: The Cartographer's Logic We cannot stick needles into every corner of the brain—that would destroy the very thing we are trying to save. Instead, we use a mathematical map to see the invisible.

This is the genius of the Kalman Filter. It operates on a principle called the Internal Model (represented mathematically as Matrix A).

Think of Matrix A as a map of the brain's gossip network. We know from pre-surgical scans that the deep brain and the surface brain are old friends—they talk constantly. If the deep brain shouts, the surface brain flinches.

Predicting the Shadow Here is how it changes the game: The Kalman filter watches the surface electrode (Node i). Suddenly, Node i twitches. It's not a seizure—just a slight, weird fluctuation. A standard machine would ignore it.

But the Kalman filter looks at its map (A). It thinks: "Node i never twitches like that unless its deep partner, Node j, is screaming."

It runs the logic backward. It infers the fire from the smoke.

The Magic of Negative Lead Time This inference creates something almost magical called negative lead time.

Old Way: We detect the seizure at T+5 seconds (after it hits the surface).

Kalman Way: We detect the seizure at T−2 seconds.

We are essentially the seismologist in London detecting the vibrations of an earthquake in Tokyo before the news even breaks. We are catching the shadow of the seizure before the seizure physically arrives. For the patient, this is the difference between being warned and being struck down.

Part II: The Symphony of Life (Sensor Fusion)

The Chaos of Living For a long time, we treated patients like batteries—we only measured their voltage (EEG).

But human beings are noisy. We chew. We run. We grit our teeth. I have spent hours cleaning data ruined by a ham sandwich. When you chew, the temporalis muscle on your temple fires. To a dumb sensor, that rhythmic muscle firing looks exactly like a seizure.

If a brain implant shocks a patient every time they eat lunch, that device isn't a cure; it's a curse.

Enter the Multimodal Shield Modern engineering acknowledges that life is messy. We now treat the patient as a complete system, using Sensor Fusion. We combine:

EEG: The speed of electricity.

Optical Sensors (NIRS): The truth of blood flow.

Accelerometers: The context of movement.

The Trust Mechanism (Matrix R) How do you get these three to agree? You use the Kalman filter's "Trust Meter," formally known as the Noise Covariance Matrix (R).

Matrix R asks a simple question moment-by-moment: "Who is lying right now?"

The Scenario: The Jogger Let's look at a patient going for a run to see this in action.

The Noise: The patient's feet hit the pavement. Their head bobs. The EEG cables jiggle, and neck muscles tense. The voltage signal goes chaotic. A standard detector screams, "Seizure!" and shocks the patient. The patient falls.

The Kalman Correction:

The Check: The system checks the Accelerometer. It sees rhythmic bouncing. It realizes: "They are running. The EEG is compromised."

The Adjustment: It dials up the noise value (REEG) for the EEG. It effectively mutes the EEG, saying, "I don't trust you right now."

The Pivot: It turns to the Optical Sensor. Seizures require a massive rush of blood to the brain. The Optical sensor says, "Blood flow is normal. No surge."

The Verdict: The filter fuses the data, weighted by trust. It ignores the noisy EEG and listens to the calm blood flow.

The device concludes: "No Seizure." The patient keeps running, unaware that a mathematical debate just happened inside their skull.

Conclusion: Reclaiming Agency

The shift from simple threshold detection to Kalman-based inference is not just a technical upgrade. It is an ethical one.

It represents a shift from viewing the brain as a black box to viewing it as a dynamic, living system.

Subtopic 10.2 gives us the eyes to see into the dark, protecting patients from the seizures they feel but cannot show.

Subtopic 10.3 gives us the wisdom to distinguish a medical emergency from a morning jog.

Ultimately, this math isn't about control. It's about freedom. It's about giving a person the confidence that their guardian angel knows the difference between a seizure and a sandwich.

The Shapeshifter: Why Our Machines Must Learn to Drift

1. The Betrayal of the Static Map

Imagine you buy a beautiful, tailored suit. It fits perfectly. You feel confident. But imagine that your body changes shape radically every single night—your arms lengthen, your posture shifts, your muscles rearrange. By Tuesday, that tailored suit is a straitjacket.

For decades, this is exactly how we treated the brain.

We viewed the brain as a rigid circuit board—a "rock." We built mathematical decoders (maps) that assumed if we calibrated a device on Monday, it would still work on Friday. We were wrong.

The brain is not a rock; it is a river. It is a biological storm of constant change. Neurons die. Synapses strengthen or fade. The physical implant shifts slightly in the gelatinous tissue of the cortex. This is non-stationarity.

2. The Tragedy of Elias

To truly feel the weight of this, let's step away from the math and look at Elias.

Elias is a patient with a high-performance intracortical array. On Day 1, we calibrate. The system is singing. Elias thinks "move up," and the cursor flies up. He feels liberated. The barrier between his mind and the world has dissolved.

Two months later, Elias returns. He tries the same mental command. The cursor jitters. It drifts diagonally. He strains, sweating, trying to force the machine to understand him.

Why?

The Hardware: Glial cells (scar tissue) have wrapped around the electrode, muffling the microphone.

The Biology: Elias's brain has learned. It has optimized its firing patterns, but our decoder is still looking for the old, clumsy patterns.

The static filter stubbornly insists: "My math is perfect; the brain is wrong." We need a filter humble enough to say: "The brain has changed; I must change with it."

3. The Solution: The Pilot and The Navigator

Enter Dual Kalman Filtering.

Think of this not as one algorithm, but as a partnership. It is like a Rally Car race. You have a Driver (the Pilot) and a Co-Driver (the Navigator).

The Pilot (State Filter):

Job: Immediate reaction.

Timescale: Milliseconds.

Question: "Where does Elias want to go right now?"

Output: Velocity, Position (x).

The Navigator (Parameter Filter):

Job: Structural analysis.

Timescale: Minutes, hours, days.

Question: "Has the map changed? Are the wheels slipping? Do we need to update our understanding of the car?"

Output: The tuning weights (A).

In a static system, only the Pilot is working. In Dual Estimation, the Navigator watches the Pilot's errors. If the Pilot consistently misses the turn, the Navigator realizes, "Wait, the steering alignment has drifted," and updates the physics of the car in real-time.

4. The Mathematics of Forgiveness

The magic of this adaptability lives in a simple concept: The Random Walk.

We take all the synaptic weights—the complex relationships between neurons—and bundle them into a vector called w. In the old days, w was a statue. In the living model, w is a traveler.

We model it like this:
$w_{k+1}=w_k+r_k$

This equation is poetic in its simplicity:

- w_{k+1}: The brain tomorrow.
- w_k: The brain today.
- r_k: The Drift (Process Noise).

Why is r_k the hero? r_k is a small random vector. It is the mathematical equivalent of permission. By adding r_k, we tell the algorithm: "I allow you to be imperfect. I expect you to be slightly different than you were a microsecond ago."

This allows the decoder to "breathe" alongside the patient. As the neural firing rates drift, the math drifts with them.

5. The Ghost in the Machine

Watching a Dual Kalman Filter (DKF) work in real-time feels eerie, almost like the machine has intuition.

A Field Note: I once watched a session where a primate subject's neural signals shifted suddenly—likely the electrode array settling deeper into the tissue. In a static system, the cursor would have crashed. Game over.

But we were running a DKF. I saw the cursor wobble for three seconds. That was the Parameter Filter waking up. It detected the mismatch, realized Neuron #42 was no longer reliable, and rewrote the weight for that neuron instantly.

The cursor snapped back to stability. The subject didn't even notice. The machine had healed itself.

Scenario	Static Filter Outcome	Dual Filter Outcome
Morning vs. Afternoon	Mental fatigue changes firing rates. Accuracy drops 20%.	Parameters slowly drift to account for fatigue. Accuracy holds.
Stroke Recovery	Brain rewires circuits. Device becomes obsolete.	Decoder "learns" the new circuits alongside the patient.

6. The Cost: Why Not Always?

You might ask, "Why don't we use this for everything?"

1. The "Overthinking" Problem: Estimating the state (intent) is cheap. Estimating the parameters (the brain's structure) is computationally expensive. If you have 100 neurons, the covariance matrix becomes massive. It used to require a rack of servers; now, thanks to the Unscented Kalman Filter, we can squeeze it onto wearable chips.

2. The Hallucination Risk: If the Navigator is too sensitive (if we make the noise term rk too big), the system becomes gullible. It starts interpreting random neural noise as meaningful structural change. It creates patterns where there are none. We have to tune the system to be "open-minded, but not naive."

7. The Fit-and-Forget Dream

The ultimate goal of Neural Engineering isn't a device that works in the lab. It's a device that works for a lifetime.

We want a pacemaker for the mind. Something you implant once and never touch again. The equation wk+1 =wk+rk is the key to that longevity.

It turns the BCI into a symbiotic companion. As the patient ages, as they learn new skills, as their brain chemistry alters, the "ghost" in the silicon evolves with them. It transforms the technology from a rigid tool into a fluid extension of the self.

The Path of Least Resistance: Optimal Control and Energy Minimization

The Art of the Neural Whisper: Teaching Machines to Listen

Imagine you are a bodyguard. Your client is a VIP (Very Important Patient). Your job is to protect them from an attacker (a Seizure).

But there is a catch: You have a gun, but you only have six bullets to last for five years.

If you fire at shadows, you run out of ammo, and your client is left defenseless. If you hesitate when the real attacker comes, your client gets hurt.

This is the heart-pounding reality of designing implantable neurotechnology. It isn't just about engineering; it is about high-stakes resource management. We are trapped between the biological imperative to cure and the physical tyranny of the battery.

The Engineer's Dilemma: Brute Force vs. The "Nudge"

In the early days of brain stimulation, we used "Brute Force." We treated the brain like a malfunctioning television—just smack it until it works. We blasted current continuously or fired aggressively at the slightest twitch.

The result?

Tissue Damage: We risked frying the very neurons we meant to save.

Battery Death: Patients faced risky surgeries every 18 months to replace exhausted generators.

We needed a smarter way. We needed a device that wasn't a "shouting match" but a "conversation." We needed the Path of Least Resistance.

Enter the Linear Quadratic Regulator (LQR). It sounds like a boring calculator, but in practice, it is a digital philosopher. It asks one profound question: What is the minimum amount of force required to achieve peace?

The "Pain Score" (The Cost Function J)

To teach a machine to be efficient, you have to give it a scoreboard. In control theory, we call this the Cost Function (J).

Think of J as a "Regret Meter." The machine wants to live a life with zero regrets. Its regret comes from two sources:

Letting the patient seize (Failure of duty).

Wasting electricity (Failure of efficiency).

Mathematically, the machine is constantly calculating this "Regret Integral" over time:
$J=\int_0^\infty (x(t)^T Q x(t)+u(t)^T R u(t))dt$

Let's translate that terrifying equation into human emotions:

x(t) (The Chaos): How far is the brain from "calm"? Is it seizing?

u(t) (The Effort): How hard is the device working? How many volts are we using?

The Goal: Keep the total J as close to zero as possible.

The Personality Test: The Battle Between Q and R

The magic of LQR lies in two matrices inside that equation: Q and R. These aren't just variables; they are the personality traits of the brain implant. We tune them to define what the device cares about.

The Q Matrix (The Helicopter Parent) Q represents how much we panic about the seizure.

High Q: "I don't care about the cost! Save the patient NOW!"

Behavior: The device becomes aggressive. It creates a "safety first" environment but drains the battery fast.

The R Matrix (The Frugal Accountant) R represents how much we value the battery.

High R: "Electricity is expensive. Do we really need to shock them? Let's wait a second."

Behavior: The device is stingy. It uses gentle nudges instead of shocks. It takes risks to save power.

The Sweet Spot: LQR is the mediator. It finds the perfect mathematical compromise between the Panic (Q) and the Frugalness (R).

Scenario	Q Setting	R Setting	Result
Life-Threatening Seizures	Very High	Low	Burn the battery. Save the life.
Mild "Auras" / Dizziness	Low	High	Tolerate minor symptoms. Save the battery for the big one.

The Solution: The "Aikido" Move (u=−Kx)

So, how does the device actually act? It uses a control law that is elegant in its simplicity:
u(t)=−KLQRx(t)

This is not an ON/OFF switch. This is a dimmer switch.

If the seizure is tiny (x is small), the zap is a whisper (u is small).

If the seizure is massive (x is large), the zap is a shout (u is large).

This is similar to the martial art of Aikido. You don't meet force with opposing force; you match the momentum. You use the minimum energy necessary to redirect the opponent. By dynamically adjusting the voltage, we stop using sledgehammers to crack nuts.

The "Oracle": The Riccati Equation

You might ask, "How does a tiny microchip inside a skull know exactly how much force to use?"

It cheats.

It uses a cheat sheet calculated before surgery using the Algebraic Riccati Equation:
ATS+SA−SBR−1BTS+Q=0

Think of the Riccati Equation as a Chess Grandmaster simulating the game millions of times before the first pawn is moved.

It studies the patient's brain (A).

It studies the device's power (B).

It looks at our priorities (Q & R).

It solves the puzzle offline, on a powerful computer, to generate the perfect strategy (K). When the device is finally implanted, it doesn't need to do complex math. It just follows the strategy. It reacts instantly.

A Tale of Two Realities: Sarah's Story

Let's look at "Sarah," a patient with temporal lobe epilepsy, to see the difference.

The Old Way (The Dumb Trigger): Sarah's device was set to trigger whenever neural activity crossed a threshold.

Monday: Sarah gets startled by a loud noise. Her brain spikes. ZAP.

Tuesday: Sarah laughs too hard. Her brain spikes. ZAP.

Wednesday: Real seizure. ZAP.

Outcome: Sarah feels anxious and "over-stimulated." Her battery dies in 2 years.

The New Way (LQR Optimal Control): Sarah gets a device tuned with LQR (High R penalty).

Monday: Startle response. The device sees the spike (x), but calculates the cost of action (R). It realizes the spike will fade naturally. Action: 0 Volts.

Tuesday: Laughter. The device watches. Action: 0 Volts.

Wednesday: A seizure begins to synchronize deep in the hippocampus. The device detects the growing error (x). It applies a precise, low-voltage counter-signal (0.5V) to destabilize the rhythm.

Outcome: The seizure dissolves before Sarah even feels it. Her battery lasts 7 years.

The Honest Truth: The Map is Not the Territory

We must end on a note of humility. LQR is beautiful, but it relies on Linearity. It assumes the brain behaves in straight lines (if 1V does X, 2V does 2X).

The brain, however, is the most chaotic, non-linear system in the universe. It is a jungle, not a highway.

If the brain changes—if Sarah ages, or her neural pathways shift—the pre-calculated map (K) might become wrong. This is why the future is Adaptive Control. We are building devices that don't just follow a map, but redraw the map every night while the patient sleeps.

Conclusion: The Restraint of Power

Optimal control teaches us a lesson that goes beyond engineering: Just because you have the power, doesn't mean you should use it.

By penalizing excess energy, we force our technology to be elegant. We force it to respect the biological tissue it inhabits. The "Path of Least Resistance" isn't about being lazy; it's about being harmonious. It is about saving the battery, yes—but ultimately, it is about saving the human.

The Diplomat and the Storm: A Human Perspective on Neural Control

Subject: Subtopics 11.2 & 11.3 | Context: The intersection of Control Theory and Biological Survival

We often approach the brain with the arrogance of an architect looking at an empty lot. We bring our blueprints (control laws), our materials (electrodes), and our power tools (stimulators), assuming we are building on passive ground.

But the brain is not an empty lot. It is a bustling, chaotic, ancient metropolis that has been running its own economy for millions of years. It has its own laws, its own currency (ATP), and its own police force (homeostasis). When we install a neural interface, we are not the builders; we are the guests. And as Section 11.2 and 11.3 reveal, if we are rude guests—if we shout too loud or move too slow—we will be evicted.

Here is the physics of that negotiation.

1. The Cost of Hesitation (Reframing Minimum Energy)

In engineering school, we solve for stability as if time is just an axis on a graph. In the brain, time is debt.

When a seizure begins, it isn't a static event; it is a compounding interest crisis. The neurons are recruiting one another into a synchronized rebellion. The equation for the Minimum Energy (Emin) required to stop this rebellion is terrifying because of what it says about procrastination.
$Emin=x0TeATTWc-1(T)eATx0$

Let's strip the academic veneer off this equation and look at the "financial" reality it describes:

The Debt (x_0): This is the seizure onset. It's the initial balance on the credit card.

The Interest Rate (e^{AT}): This is the killer. Because the eigenvalues of a seizure are positive (unstable), the "interest" on the debt grows exponentially. Every millisecond you wait, the cost to pay it back doubles, then triples.

The Liquidity (W_c^{-1}): The Inverse Gramian represents how hard it is to move money around. If the brain is in a "stiff" state (singular Gramian), you have no liquidity. You have to pay a massive premium to change the state.

The Whisper vs. The Scream

The "Avalanche Effect" implies a profound design philosophy: The Whisper Strategy.

If our detection algorithms are fast enough ($T \approx 0$), we can stop a seizure with a "whisper"—a micro-stimulation so subtle the patient never feels it. We pay off the debt while it's still pennies.

But if we wait for the "Aura" (clinical symptoms)—if we wait until the patient feels the fear—we are too late. The boulder is already at the bottom of the hill. To stop it now, we have to scream (high-current stimulation). We have to slam the brakes. And as we see in the next section, slamming the brakes leaves skid marks on the biology.

2. The Bankruptcy of the Cell (Metabolic Cost)

Section 11.3 moves us from the battery of the device to the "battery" of the cell.

The brain is an elitist organ. It weighs 2% of the body but demands 20% of the lunch. It lives on a razor's edge of energy supply. Every time a neuron fires, it spends gold (ATP) to reset its pumps.

We can model the brain’s survival instinct as an internal LQR controller trying to minimize this cost function:
$J=\int_0^\infty (x^T Q_{bio} x + u^T R_{bio} u)dt$

The term $u^T R_{bio} u$ is the brain's way of saying: "Do not make me work harder than I have to."

The "Backseat Driver" Problem

Here is the tragedy of poor engineering: We often design devices that act like a panicked backseat driver. Imagine the brain (the driver) detects a slide (seizure). Its natural instinct is to release GABA (pump the brakes). If our device detects the same slide and decides to slam the steering wheel in the opposite direction (depolarization block), we aren't helping. We are fighting the driver.

This creates Metabolic Friction. We force the neurons to fire when they want to rest, or rest when they want to fire. We deplete their ATP reserves.

The pumps fail.

The ion gradients collapse.

Calcium floods the cell like water into a sinking ship.

The cell doesn't just die; it undergoes excitotoxicity. It is chemically digested from the inside out. We "controlled" the voltage, but we bankrupted the biology.

3. The Art of "Judo" Control (The Synthesis)

The future of neural interfaces isn't about being stronger than the seizure; it's about being smarter than the dynamics.

We are moving toward Biomimetic Control. This is the engineering equivalent of Judo. In Judo, you don't stop an opponent by standing in front of them (High Energy). You stop them by using their own momentum to tip them off balance (Minimum Energy).

By tuning our device matrices (Qdevice, Rdevice) to harmonize with the brain's internal matrices (Qbio, Rbio), we stop fighting the current.

Old Way: Detect seizure → Blast with electricity.

New Way: Detect the trajectory toward seizure → Apply a subtle nudge orthogonal to the flow → Watch the brain's own homeostatic mechanisms slide the state back to stability.

The Human Conclusion

The math of the Inverse Gramian and the Metabolic Cost function tells us a story of empathy.

11.2 tells us to be attentive. Watch the system closely so you can intervene with a whisper, not a shout.

11.3 tells us to be respectful. Acknowledge that the tissue has a limited budget, and do not spend what the patient cannot afford.

True neural engineering is not about domination. It is about partnership. It is the search for the minimum energy required to restore the maximum amount of life.

The Art of Neural Silence: A Manifesto for Sparse Control

Subtopic 11.4: Sparsity Constraints (LASSO)

In neural engineering, we are often seduced by the power of our own hardware. We build chips with 64, 128, or 1,000 channels, and our instinct is to use them all. But the human brain does not speak in "walls of sound." It speaks in precise, sparse firing patterns.

When we blast the brain with "dense" control signals (activating every electrode simultaneously), we aren't just being mathematically lazy; we are being biologically reckless. This is the story of why Sparsity—the art of doing more with less—is the most critical safety feature in modern neural interfaces.

I. The Villain: The "Greedy" Regulator (LQR)

To understand the solution, we must first understand the trap. The industry standard for control is the Linear Quadratic Regulator (LQR).

LQR is a mathematical "people pleaser." Its cost function relies on the L2 Norm (squaring the numbers). Because of the geometry of squares, LQR hates "big" numbers. It would much rather give 10 electrodes a tiny voltage of 0.1V than give 1 electrode a strong voltage of 1.0V.

J=Σ (xTQx+uTRu)

The Result? The "Shotgun" Effect. The LQR controller activates all 32 electrodes on your implant at a low hum.

In Silicon: This is fine. The chip handles it.

In the Brain: It is a disaster. It creates a "muddy" electrical field where current leaks everywhere. It heats up the tissue. It drains the battery in months.

The Insight: LQR creates a "noisy room" where everyone is whispering. We need a controller that acts like a single person speaking clearly into a microphone.

II. The Hero: The Geometry of Diamonds (LASSO)

To fix this, we change the rules of the game. We stop punishing the square of the input and start punishing the absolute value. This is the L1 Penalty, commonly known as LASSO.

$$J=\sum_{k=0}^{N}(x_k^T Q x_k+\lambda \| u_k \|_1)$$

Why does this simple change silence the noise? It comes down to geometry.

The "Pointy" Intuition Imagine you are blowing up a balloon inside a box.

L2 (The Circle): The balloon hits the smooth wall of a circle. It touches at a weird angle, giving you values like 0.32 or 0.15. Nothing is zero.

L1 (The Diamond): The constraint shape is a diamond with sharp corners that lie perfectly on the axes. When the optimizer minimizes cost, it "snags" on these sharp corners.

The Consequence: Because the corners are on the axes, the solution for most electrodes becomes exactly zero. The math forces the controller to pick the 2 or 3 "MVP" electrodes and kill the power to the other 29.

III. The Hardware Reality: Why "Zero" Saves Lives

Why do we fight so hard for these zeros? Because in the wet, salty environment of the human body, "Off" is the most valuable state.

1. The Heat Problem

Neural tissue is incredibly fragile. A temperature rise of just 1°C can cause irreversible tissue damage.

Dense Control: 32 current sources running simultaneously generate heat both at the chip (in the chest/skull) and at the electrode tip.

Sparse Control: Only 2 sources are active. The thermal footprint is negligible.

2. The "Greyout" (Retinal Implants)

Imagine a blind patient with a retinal implant. They are looking at a door frame.

Without Sparsity: The controller tries to draw the door using all 1,000 electrodes. Current spreads laterally. The patient sees a blurry grey fog.

With Sparsity: The LASSO controller picks the 50 pixels that define the edge of the door. The patient sees crisp points of light (phosphenes). The image is lower resolution, but it is understandable.

3. Battery Anxiety

Every time you switch a transistor, you pay a "tax" in power. A dense control vector is a battery vampire. Sparse control extends the recharge cycle from days to weeks, giving the patient their life back.

IV. Clinical Precision: The Sniper Approach

The most profound impact of sparsity is in Deep Brain Stimulation (DBS).

In the brain, millimeters matter. If you are stimulating the Subthalamic Nucleus for Parkinson's, your target is the size of a peanut. Just next to it is the Internal Capsule. If you hit that, the patient's face might contort, or they might slur their speech.

The LQR Blob: Creates a spherical field that spills over into danger zones.

The LASSO Beam: By driving only specific contacts hard (Current Steering), we shape the electrical field directionally. We can steer the current away from side effects and into the therapeutic target.

V. How to Engineer It (The Cheat Code)

Implementing pure L1 optimization on a tiny, low-power brain implant is hard because the absolute value function is "pointy" (non-differentiable). We can't use standard calculus.

Engineers use a brilliant hack called Iterative Reweighted LQR:

Run a standard LQR pass.

Look at the result. If Electrode 5 is barely being used (e.g., 0.01V), we assume it's useless.

Punish it. We drastically increase the "cost" (Price) of using Electrode 5 in the next round.

Run LQR again. The controller sees the high price and decides to turn Electrode 5 completely off.

After 3 loops, the system naturally converges to a sparse, efficient solution without needing a supercomputer in the chest.

Summary: The New Standard

Feature	The Old Way (LQR/L2)	The New Way (LASSO/L1)
Philosophy	The Shotgun (Hit everything a little)	The Sniper (Hit one thing perfectly)
Math Shape	Circle (Smooth)	Diamond (Pointy)
Battery Life	Drains quickly	Efficient / Long-lasting
Patient Vision	Blurry / Washed out	High Contrast / Crisp
Safety	High risk of heating	Thermally Safe

The Bottom Line: In neural engineering, silence is not empty. Silence is precision. By forcing our algorithms to be thrifty, we build interfaces that respect the biological limits of the human host.

Closing the Loop: Feedback Control Algorithms

Subtopic 12.1: Taming the Chaos – The Discrete PID Controller

1. The Great Conversation Shift: From Monologue to Dialogue

For a long time, treating the brain with electricity was like having a conversation where you do all the talking and never listen. We call this Open-Loop stimulation. We would implant an electrode and blast the brain with a constant "noise" (e.g., 130 Hz, 3 Volts) regardless of whether the patient was sleeping, running a marathon, or having a panic attack. It was a monologue. It worked, but it was blunt, inefficient, and often created side effects because we were shouting when we should have been whispering.

Closed-Loop control changes the dynamic. It turns the monologue into a dialogue. We stop shouting. We listen first.

The PID Controller is the translator in this dialogue. It listens to the brain's internal state and calculates exactly how much electricity is needed to nudge the patient back to health—no more, no less. It is 19th-century steam engine math adapted for the 21st-century human mind.

2. The Target: Finding "The Goldilocks Zone"

Before we control anything, we need to know what we are looking for. In a thermostat, the error is a temperature difference. In the brain, the "error" is a pathological rhythm.

Take Parkinson's Disease. A healthy brain has a flexible, chaotic rhythm. A Parkinsonian brain gets stuck in a synchronized marching beat called the Beta Band (13–30 Hz). This rigidity causes the tremors and stiffness patients feel.

We define our variables like this:

The Setpoint ($r[k]$): The "Goldilocks" zone. We want the Beta power low (healthy).

The Reality ($y[k]$): The current Beta power we are actually recording.

The Error ($e[k]$): The gap between the two.

$$e[k]=y[k]-r[k]$$

If $e[k]$ is zero, the brain is healthy, and the controller can relax. If $e[k]$ is high, the controller needs to wake up.

3. The Recipe: Slicing Time

Biological time flows like a river (continuous), but computers think in snapshots (discrete). Our microchips wake up, take a measurement, make a decision, and sleep again, thousands of times a second. We don't talk about time t; we talk about the sample step k.

Here is the "brain" of the controller—the Discrete PID Formula:

$$u[k]=Kpe[k]+Kij=0\Sigma ke[j]\Delta t+Kd\Delta te[k]-e[k-1]$$

It looks intimidating, but it is actually just three distinct personalities arguing over how to drive the car.

The Three Personalities

P: The Proportional Term (Kp) – "The Panic Button"

This term lives entirely in the Present. It looks at the error right now and reacts instantly.

The Philosophy: "The house is on fire right now? Pour water on it right now!"

The Risk: If Kp is too low, the tremor never stops. If Kp is too high, the system panics. It pushes too hard, the brain fights back, and you end up causing oscillations—literally shaking the brain with electricity.

I: The Integral Term (Ki) – "The Historian"

This term lives in the Past. It keeps a running tally (sum) of every error that has ever happened.

The Philosophy: "I noticed that for the last 10 minutes, your Proportional panic wasn't enough to stop the tremor. There is a stubborn, steady-state error remaining. I am going to slowly ramp up the pressure until that last bit of tremor is crushed."

The Value: The "P" term gets you close; the "I" term gets you to perfection.

D: The Derivative Term (Kd) – "The Fortune Teller"

This term lives in the Future. It looks at the rate of change ($e[k]-e[k-1]$).

The Philosophy: "Whoa, slow down! The tremor is dropping rapidly. If you keep stimulating this hard, you're going to overshoot the target. I'm hitting the brakes before we crash."

The Danger: In the lab, we are terrified of the D-term. Why? Noise.

If a patient sneezes, the electrical signal spikes. The Derivative term sees this massive spike, thinks the world is ending, and slams the stimulation to maximum voltage. Because of this, we usually keep the D-term turned off or heavily filtered in neural applications.

4. Engineering "In the Wild": When Math Meets Biology

Writing the equation is easy; keeping a patient safe is hard. Here are the "gotchas" that don't show up in textbooks but keep engineers awake at night.

The "Sticky Gas Pedal" (Integrator Windup)

Imagine you are stopped at a red light, but you keep pressing the gas pedal harder and harder. The car doesn't move (because of the brakes), but the engine is roaring. When the light turns green, you will launch into traffic at 100 mph.

This is Integrator Windup.

The tremor is severe.

The "I-term" (Historian) asks for more voltage: 4V... 5V... 10V... 20V.

The battery is physically limited to 5V. It can't give more.

But the math keeps counting up to 20V.

Suddenly, the tremor stops. The error is zero. The stimulation should drop.

But the Historian remembers "20V." It takes forever to count back down, roasting the patient's brain with max voltage when they don't need it.

The Fix: We use Clamping. We tell the math: "If the battery is maxed out, stop counting."

The "Washout" Effect (The Rubber Band)

Biology fights back. I once worked on a system where the PID controller worked perfectly—it suppressed the pathological signal completely. But when we turned the device off to save battery, the brain didn't just return to normal; it rebounded. The symptoms came back worse than before.

The brain had adapted to the constant pressure of the Integral term. When that pressure was removed, the brain snapped back like a stretched rubber band. We learned that sometimes, "perfect" control is too aggressive. We have to be gentle.

5. The Dark Art of Tuning

In industrial robotics, you tune a PID controller by pushing it until the system vibrates, then backing off (Ziegler-Nichols method).

You cannot do this in a human brain. Making a brain vibrate can trigger a seizure.

We use Heuristic "Safe" Tuning:

Kill the Memory: Set Ki and Kd to zero.

Nudge the Present: Slowly increase Kp until the symptoms drop by about 50%.

Add the Memory: Slowly introduce Ki to wipe up the remaining symptoms.

Ignore the Future: Leave Kd at zero unless absolutely necessary to dampen aggressive spikes.

Key Takeaway: In 90% of neural interfaces, a PI (Proportional-Integral) controller is the gold standard. The Derivative term is often too risky given how noisy biological data is.

6. Summary

The Discrete PID controller (u[k]) is the workhorse of modern bio-electronic medicine. It replaces "blind" stimulation with an intelligent, reactive loop. However, it requires a deep respect for the hardware. You aren't controlling a steam valve; you are controlling a neural network that adapts, fights back, and is full of noise.

The next evolution? Model Predictive Control (MPC). PID is reactive (fixing errors after they happen). MPC is predictive (fixing errors before they happen). But for now, PID remains the reliable bridge between silicon and neurons.

Subtopic 12.2: Tuning Gains for Neural Dynamics & Subtopic 12.3: Model Predictive Control (MPC)

Introduction: The Edge of Chaos

To understand neural control, you must first abandon the idea that the brain is a computer. A computer is deterministic; if you press 'A', you get 'A'. The brain, however, is a biological storm. It operates on the "Edge of Criticality"—a metastable tightrope walk where billions of neurons hum in a chaotic harmony.

In epilepsy, this harmony collapses. The brain slides from complex, healthy chaos into a rhythmic, shouting unison—a seizure.

As engineers, our job isn't just to build a circuit; it is to build an Artificial Reflex. We are trying to stabilize a system that is actively trying to run away from us. We are balancing a pencil on a fingertip, but the pencil is made of jelly, and the lights in the room are flickering.

We have two main philosophies for this task: the reactive brawler (PID) and the calculating grandmaster (MPC).

Subtopic 12.2: The PID Framework (The Artificial Instinct)

The PID controller is the "Old Reliable" of engineering. It powers your thermostat and your car's cruise control. But when we wire it into the human cortex, it stops being a simple equation and becomes a surrogate nervous system. It creates a synthetic reflex loop designed to punch back when the brain misbehaves.

I. The Proportional Gain (Kp): The Knee-Jerk Reaction

Think of Kp as the controller's muscle. It operates on a simple, brutish logic: "The bigger the error, the harder I hit."

If the neural activity spikes (the error $e(t)$ grows), the Proportional term commands a massive surge of current:
$u(t)=Kp \cdot e(t)$

The "Ghost in the Machine" (Delay-Induced Instability)
Tuning Kp is a white-knuckle experience. Why? Because

the brain has lag. Synapses take milliseconds to fire; hardware takes microseconds to process.

If you set Kp too high, you fall into the trap of the delayed reflex. Imagine trying to catch a falling glass while wearing video goggles that are delayed by half a second. You see the glass fall, you snatch at it, but it's already gone. Worse, your snatch knocks over a second glass. In the brain, this is called "Ringing." The stimulation arrives too late, hitting the neurons when they are trying to rest, inadvertently pumping energy into the seizure rather than suppressing it.

The Safety Circle (Z-Transform) We visualize this danger zone using the Z-plane. We draw a "Unit Circle" ($|z|=1$). As we crank up the gain Kp, the system's "poles" (instability markers) drift outward. The moment a pole crosses that circle, the controller itself becomes the seizure generator. We tune for the "sweet spot"—strong enough to fight, weak enough to listen.

II. The Integral Term (Ki): The Grudge Holder

If Kp is a reflex, Ki is a memory. It doesn't care about right now; it cares about the past.
$u(t)=K_i \int_0^t e(\tau)d\tau$

Battling the Slow Drift Seizures often have a "pre-ictal" phase—a slow, creeping drift in potassium or background voltage that suggests a storm is brewing. The Proportional term is too dumb to notice this subtle drift. But the Integral term watches the error accumulate. It realizes, "Hey, we've been slightly off-balance for ten minutes," and slowly ramps up the pressure to nudge the brain back to safety.

The Danger: Integral Windup The risk is that the Integral term holds a grudge. If the brain is stubborn and doesn't fix itself, Ki keeps adding pressure, ramping the voltage higher and higher until it hits the battery's limit. When the brain finally relaxes, Ki is still "wound up," screaming at full volume at a now-calm brain. We have to program "anti-windup" logic—essentially telling the controller to take a deep breath and let it go.

III. The Derivative Term (Kd): The Paranoid Oracle

The Derivative term attempts to predict the future by looking at the speed of the error.
u(t)=Kddtde(t)

The Preemptive Strike Kd is the only part of the PID loop that acts before the disaster. If it sees the neural signal rocket upward, it slams the brakes immediately, even if the seizure hasn't technically started yet.

The Noise Problem The problem is that Kd is paranoid. To a derivative term, a tiny, harmless pop of static noise looks exactly like the start of a massive seizure because the slope is vertical. Without sunglasses—specifically, a Low-Pass Filter to block high-frequency noise—the Derivative term will shock the patient every time a neuron hiccups.

Subtopic 12.3: Model Predictive Control (The Chess Grandmaster)

If PID is a driver reacting to brake lights ahead, Model Predictive Control (MPC) is a GPS system that sees the traffic jam five miles away and reroutes you before you even see it.

MPC represents a paradigm shift from Reaction to Optimization.

I. The Philosophy: Playing the Movie Forward

PID is blind; it only knows what is happening now. MPC is visionary. It holds a mathematical map of the patient's brain (State-Space Model):

$$x_{k+1}=Ax_k+Bu_k$$

It asks a profound question: "Based on my model of this specific brain, what sequence of shocks over the next 100ms will result in the best outcome?"

II. The Cost Function: The Budget Negotiation

MPC doesn't just "fix" the error. It balances a checkbook. It solves a massive optimization problem (J) at every time step, weighing two competing desires:

- The State Penalty (x^TQx): We want the seizure to stop (Error = 0).
- The Control Penalty (u^TRu): We want to save battery and spare the tissue.

$$J=\sum_{i=0}^{N-1}\left(x_{k+i}^TQx_{k+i}+u_{k+i}^TRu_{k+i}\right)$$

This equation is a negotiation.

- Q is the fear of seizures.
- R is the frugality of the engineer. If we set R high, the controller becomes a miser, only stimulating if absolutely necessary. It realizes that blasting the brain with 5 Volts is "expensive" (tissue damage, battery drain) and calculates the minimum effective dose to derail the seizure.

III. The Receding Horizon: Correcting the Map

The genius of MPC is that it doesn't trust its own long-term plan.

It calculates the best move for the next 10 steps.

It executes only step 1.

Then, it throws the rest of the plan away, looks at the brain again, and re-calculates.
This is the Receding Horizon. Because the brain is chaotic and our models are imperfect, the "traffic" changes. By re-planning every millisecond, MPC constantly corrects for the "plant mismatch"—the gap between our math and biological reality.

IV. Handling Constraints: The Reality Check

PID tries to be a hero; if the error is huge, it demands infinite voltage. The hardware clips it, and the PID math breaks down.
MPC is a realist. We explicitly program the constraints:
$|u_k| \leqslant I_{max}$
MPC knows it only has 5 Volts. It won't waste time wishing for 100 Volts. Instead, it finds the most clever, efficient way to use the 5 Volts it has. It doesn't panic; it strategizes within its limits.

Summary: The Bifurcation
PID is the reflex arc. It is fast, cheap, and visceral. It feels the error and pushes back.
MPC is the frontal cortex. It plans, predicts, and budgets. As we move toward smarter implants, we are drifting from the reflex of PID to the foresight of MPC, treating the epileptic brain not just as a nail to be hammered, but as a dynamic landscape to be navigated.

Finding the Target: Source Localization and Inverse Problems

The Ghost in the Machine: Solving the Inverse Problem

1. The Impossible Ask: Plato's Cave with Electrodes

Imagine you are standing outside a massive, soundproof concert hall. The walls are thick concrete (the skull). You cannot see the band. You cannot hear the music clearly. All you have are 19 vibration sensors (electrodes) taped to the outer walls.

Suddenly, the sensors vibrate.

Your job is to answer two questions: Who played that note? And where are they standing?

This is the Inverse Problem. We have the "effect" (voltage on the scalp), but we are desperate for the "cause" (current density in the brain).

In the world of pure mathematics, this is called an "ill-posed" problem. Why? Because a tiny whisper right next to the wall (scalp) produces the exact same vibration as a massive scream from the center of the room (deep brain). There are infinite combinations of internal energy that could create the map we see on the surface.

To solve an impossible math problem, we have to cheat. We have to introduce bias. We have to tell the computer: "Don't just give me any answer that fits the math. Give me the answer that fits Biology."

2. The LORETA Philosophy: From Dots to Clouds

In the early days, we treated the brain like a simple physics diagram. We used "Dipole Fitting." We assumed that a seizure or a thought was a single, tiny dot—a specific point in space firing off energy.

But the brain is not a collection of isolated dots. It is a wet, living network.

LORETA (Low-Resolution Brain Electromagnetic Tomography) changed the paradigm by introducing a simple, beautiful biological truth: The brain is smooth.

The Neighbor Rule: If a neuron at location X is screaming, the neurons at location X+1 are likely screaming too.

The Weather Map: Brain activity shouldn't look like a starry sky (random, sharp pinpoints of light). It should look like a weather map (gradients of high and low pressure).

LORETA solves the Inverse Problem by forcing the solution to be blurred. It looks for the smoothest possible distribution of energy that still explains the data.

3. Under the Hood: The Mathematics of Empathy

To find the source (J), we look at the voltages (V). The relationship is linear, but getting back to the source requires a complex filter.

The estimation of the source current is derived from this transformation matrix T:

$$T=W-1KT(KW-1KT+aH)-1$$

This formula looks cold, but every variable represents a specific physical or "emotional" struggle in the lab. Let's humanize the components.

A. The Lead Field Matrix (K): The Terrain Map

Think of K as the Passport. It contains the physics of the specific patient's head.

It knows how thick the skull is.

It knows where the brain folds (gyri) and dips (sulci).

It calculates the cost of travel.

If electricity travels from the deep hippocampus to the frontal electrode, K dictates exactly how much signal is lost along the way. If your K is wrong (e.g., using a generic head model for a patient with a skull defect), the map is useless.

B. The Weighting Matrix (W): The Equity Officer

This is the most critical part for "fairness" in the brain. Physics is unfair to deep structures. Signal strength drops off with the square of the distance (1/r2). A massive seizure in the amygdala (deep) looks like a tiny whisper by the time it hits the scalp.

Without the Weighting Matrix (W), the math is lazy. The algorithm will always dump the activity on the surface of the cortex because it requires less energy to explain the data there.

What W does: It boosts the volume of the deep sources. It tells the algorithm, "Hey, pay attention to the guys in the back of the room; they are quieter, but they might be the ones screaming."

C. The Regularization Parameter (a): The Trust Knob

Data is never perfect. Muscles twitch, lights hum, patients blink. We call this noise. a (Alpha) is our Skepticism Dial.

High a: "I don't trust this data. It's noisy. Blur the image. Ignore the sharp spikes. Give me the general 'gist' of what's happening."

Low a: "This data is pristine. Trust every tiny wiggle. If the math says the source is spiking, believe it."

Finding the right a is an art form. Set it too high, and you smudge the temporal lobe into the frontal lobe. Set it too low, and you chase ghosts—phantom sources created by random noise.

4. The Clinical Reality: Reading the Shadows

When we use this for epilepsy surgery, the "cool math" becomes terrifyingly real. We are looking for the "seizure onset zone"—the place the surgeon needs to cut out.

The Problem of the "Ghost"

LORETA images are seductive. You see a bright red blob on a 3D MRI, and your brain wants to believe "X Marks the Spot." But we must remember: This is a model, not a photograph.

Smearing: Because LORETA enforces smoothness, a pinpoint tumor seizure will look like a large cloud. We can find the center of the cloud, but we can't be sure of its edges.

Displacement: If a seizure happens deep in a fissure (a crack between brain folds), the magnetic field is oriented strangely. LORETA might project the source a few centimeters away to the nearest surface.

The Evolution: sLORETA and eLORETA

Because of these "ghosting" errors, the field evolved.

sLORETA (Standardized): This was a breakthrough. It normalizes the current by the expected noise. In perfect simulations, it has zero localization error. It is like putting glasses on the algorithm—suddenly, the blurry cloud snaps into a focused point.

eLORETA (Exact): The modern refinement, further reducing "ghost" sources and interference.

Summary

Solving the Inverse Problem is like trying to reconstruct a face based solely on its shadow. It shouldn't be possible.

But by using LORETA, we apply the biological rules of "smoothness" and "depth weighting" to narrow down the infinite possibilities to the most probable reality. It allows us to peer inside the electric storm of the human mind without ever breaking the skin.

Subtopic 13.2: The Ghost in the Machine (The Non-Uniqueness Challenge)

The "Locked Room" Mystery

In neuroengineering, we face a frustrating physical reality: the skull. While it is excellent for protecting the brain, it is terrible for listening to it. We call the skull the "ultimate low-pass filter" because it acts like a thick, soundproof wall. It muffles the sharp, crisp conversations of neurons, leaving us with only a dull, rhythmic hum on the scalp.

This creates the Inverse Problem.

Imagine you are standing outside a massive, rowdy stadium. You can hear the roar of the crowd (the EEG signal on the scalp), but your job is to identify exactly which person in Section 42, Row C, Seat 5 screamed "Goal!"

Mathematically, this is impossible to solve with certainty. This is known as Helmholtz Reciprocity.

The Hard Truth: For every pattern of electricity we record on the scalp, there are mathematically infinite combinations of brain activity that could have caused it.

It is like seeing a shadow of a hand on a wall. Is it a hand? A cardboard cutout? A strange tree branch? You cannot know for sure just by looking at the shadow. You have to make assumptions.

The "Optimist" Approach: LORETA

To solve this impossible math problem, we introduced LORETA (Low-Resolution Electromagnetic Tomography).

Think of LORETA as the "Optimist." It relies on the biological assumption of peer pressure. It assumes that neurons are conformists; if one neuron is shouting, its neighbors are likely shouting too. LORETA looks for the smoothest possible solution that explains the data.

The Flaw: While LORETA makes beautiful, smooth 3D maps, it has a "Depth Bias."

The Problem: Electricity gets weaker as it travels (Inverse Square Law). A giant scream deep in the brain sounds the same as a whisper right next to the skull.

The Error: LORETA is lazy. It prefers to explain a signal as a weak whisper on the surface rather than a scream deep inside. It often misses deep sources (like the hippocampus) entirely, painting them as a smear on the surface.

In epilepsy surgery, this is dangerous. You don't want to remove the "whispering" surface tissue if the "screaming" culprit is actually deep underneath.

The "Truth Teller": sLORETA

Enter sLORETA (Standardized LORETA). This isn't just an upgrade; it's a change in philosophy.

If LORETA looks at raw power, sLORETA looks at statistical probability. It asks not "How loud is this signal?" but "How loud is this signal compared to the noise we expect here?"

It uses a process called Variance Normalization:
J^sLORETA=J^lT[Var]−1J^l

In Plain English: Deep sources have high uncertainty (high variance). sLORETA takes the estimated activity and divides it by that uncertainty.

If a source is deep and fuzzy, sLORETA tightens the focus.

It cancels out the "Depth Bias."

The Result: sLORETA provides Zero Localization Error. This doesn't mean the image is perfect HD quality—it is still a bit blurry (low resolution). But, the center of that blur is exactly where the source is. If the seizure is in the hippocampus, sLORETA puts the red "hotspot" right on the hippocampus.

Subtopic 13.3: The "Time-Travel" Cheat (Real-Time Implementation)

The Engineering Crisis

Here is the bottleneck: Solving the math above (Inverse Problems, matrices, regularization) takes a powerful desktop computer about 50 milliseconds per frame.

The Constraint: An implanted brain chip for epilepsy (closed-loop) needs to detect a seizure and zap it in under 10 milliseconds. And it has to run on a battery the size of a coin. We cannot fit a supercomputer inside a human head.

The "Fixed Geometry" Hack

We solve this by "cheating." We realize that the stage doesn't change:

The Brain Anatomy is constant.

The Electrode Screws don't move.

The Skull Thickness is static.

Because the physics don't change, the relationship between the sensor voltage (V) and the source current (J) is linear. We can pre-calculate all the heavy math—all the calculus, the sLORETA weights, and the physics—before the patient even wakes up from surgery.

The Pipeline: "Baking the Cake"

Offline (The Lab Supercomputer): We take the MRI and electrode locations. We spend hours churning through the complex matrix inversions. We condense all that physics into a single, static Projection Matrix (T).

The Upload: We flash this Matrix T onto the tiny chip implanted in the skull.

Online (Inside the Patient): The chip is simple. It doesn't know physics. It just does multiplication.

The chip runs this simple equation every millisecond:
J^=T·V

Where:

T is our pre-baked map.

V is the raw voltage from the sensors.

This turns a complex physics problem into a simple calculator problem, allowing us to track brain activity in microseconds.

The Superpower: "Virtual Electrodes"

This math gives us a superpower: X-Ray Vision.

Usually, to see deep into the brain (like the Amygdala), you have to shove a physical needle into it. That causes damage. With the Projection Matrix, we use the surface sensors to mathematically "beam form" our focus deep into the brain. We create a Virtual Electrode.

Why is this vital?

Artifact Rejection: If the patient clenches their jaw, surface electrodes go crazy with muscle noise.

The Filter: The Projection Matrix knows that "jaw muscle noise" doesn't look like a brain signal. It spatially filters it out. The Virtual Electrode deep in the brain stays steady, ignoring the muscle noise, waiting only for the true seizure.

It transforms "dumb" sensors into an "intelligent" 3D seizure detector.

Key Takeaways for the Neuroengineer

The Shadow Problem: You can never be 100% sure what created a scalp signal, so you must use priors (assumptions).

sLORETA is the Standard: It normalizes for noise, allowing us to see deep brain sources without them getting washed out by surface activity.

The Pre-Calc Trick: We do the heavy math once on a desktop so the implant can run lightweight multiplication in real-time.

Virtual Electrodes: We can monitor deep brain structures without physically penetrating them, drastically reducing surgical risk.

Subtopic 13.4: The Sniper vs. The Floodlight

A Tale of Two Mathematical Philosophies in the Epilepsy Ward

Imagine you are standing in a dark room. On the wall, you see a shadow of a hand making a bunny rabbit. Your job is to determine—with life-or-death precision—where the hand is, how big it is, and the exact angle of the light source.

This is the Inverse Problem in EEG. The electrical squiggles on the scalp are just shadows. The "hand" is a cluster of neurons misfiring deep in the brain.

In epilepsy surgery, we aren't just guessing; we are drawing a map for a neurosurgeon. If we point to the wrong spot, healthy brain tissue gets cut, and the seizures continue. To solve this, we use two mathematical personalities: Beamforming and LORETA.

They don't just calculate differently; they think differently.

Part 1: The Beamformer (The Sniper)

Beamforming (specifically Linearly Constrained Minimum Variance, or LCMV) is the "special ops" agent of brain mapping. It is precise, arrogant, and obsessed with silence.

Its philosophy is simple: "Ignore everything except the target."

Imagine a crowded cocktail party. You are trying to listen to one person whispering in the corner. A Beamformer builds a mathematical ear trumpet that points exactly at that corner while actively building sound-proof walls to block out the laughter, clinking glasses, and chatter from the rest of the room.

The Weapon of Choice

The Beamformer uses a specific equation to build this filter. It looks intimidating, but it is actually a recipe for noise cancellation:
wbeam=(KTC−1K)−1KTC−1

Let's translate this from "Math" to "Human":

wbeam (The Scope): This is the final setting we dial in to see the target voxel (brain pixel).

K (The Map): The Lead Field. This is the physics of the patient's head. It asks, "If the target shouts, what does it sound like?"

C (The Crowd): The Data Covariance. This represents the noise of the party right now.

C−1 (The Silencer): This is the magic—and the danger. By inverting the covariance, the algorithm aggressively hunts down loud, interfering noises and deletes them.

The Fatal Flaw: The "Uncorrelated" Assumption

Beamformers are geniuses, but they are paranoid. They assume that every person at the party is having a distinct, private conversation. They assume sources are uncorrelated.

If Source A (the target) and Source B (the interference) are doing completely different things, the Beamformer works perfectly. It kills B to hear A.

Part 2: The Crash (When the Math Breaks)

Here is the tragedy of using a Sniper to hunt a Seizure.

Epilepsy is not a private conversation. It is a riot.

During a seizure, neurons aren't acting independently. They are locking arms and chanting in unison. This is called hypersynchrony. Often, a spot in the left brain will fire in perfect sync with a spot in the right brain (a "mirror focus").

The Correlation Trap:

The Beamformer looks at the Target (Left Brain).

It notices the Right Brain is doing the exact same thing at the exact same time.

The algorithm panics. Its job is to minimize total noise.

It thinks: "Wait! If I subtract the Right signal from the Left signal, the noise goes to zero!"

Result: It cancels out the seizure.

The Irony: The smarter the math tries to be (using that C^{-1} term), the more it treats the seizure as "noise" to be removed. You stare at the screen, knowing the patient is having a seizure, but the map shows... nothing. Silence.

Part 3: LORETA (The Floodlight)

If the Beamformer is a Sniper, LORETA (Low Resolution Electromagnetic Tomography) is a Floodlight—or perhaps a grand Impressionist painter.

LORETA doesn't try to filter out the noise. It doesn't scan point-by-point. It turns the lights on in the whole room at once.

The Philosophy of "Smoothness"

The Inverse Problem has infinite solutions. To pick the best one, LORETA relies on a biological truth: The brain is gooey.

It assumes that brain activity doesn't happen in single, isolated pixels. It spreads. If one neuron is shouting, its neighbors are probably whispering. LORETA forces the mathematical solution to be smooth (minimizing the Laplacian).

Why LORETA Survives the Riot

Because LORETA doesn't use that aggressive "Silencer" (C−1) to cancel out interference, it is immune to the Correlation Trap.

Synchrony? No problem.

Mirror Foci? It sees them both.

The Trade-off: The image is blurry. It's "Low Resolution" by name and nature. You get a blob, not a dot.

But in epilepsy, a blurry truth is better than a precise lie.

Part 4: The Showdown (The Toolkit)

To help you decide which tool to pull from the belt, I've broken them down by personality:
Feature The Sniper (Beamforming/LCMV) The Floodlight (LORETA/sLORETA)

Superpower Pinpoint accuracy. Can separate two sources that are 1cm apart. Reliability. It never accidentally deletes the signal.
Kryptonite Synchrony. If sources talk to each other (correlation), the math self-destructs. Blur. The solution is smeared. It's hard to tell the surgeon exactly where the edge is.
Best Used For Focal tasks (tapping a finger), sensory spikes, small lesions. Seizures (Ictal data). Tracking networks that span across the brain.
The Risk False Negatives (Missing the seizure entirely). Poor Localization (Pointing to a general area rather than a specific spot).

Part 5: Authentic Case Studies

Let's apply this to the messy reality of the clinic.

Case A: The "Mirror" Nightmare

The Patient: A child with temporal lobe epilepsy. The EEG shows spikes on the Left and Right sides at the exact same time.

Beamformer's Attempt: It sees the Left and Right signals as identical copies. It assumes one is an artifact of the other. It subtracts them. The resulting image shows a ghost spot in the center of the head (where there is no brain). Failure.

LORETA's Attempt: It paints a large, warm glow over both temporal lobes. It's not precise, but it correctly tells the doctor: "This is a bilateral network." Success.

Case B: The "Click"

The Patient: A small localized dysplasia (scar tissue) that fires sharp, random electrical pops.

LORETA's Attempt: It smears the activity across the whole parietal lobe. The surgeon asks, "Where do I cut?" and LORETA shrugs. Frustration.

Beamformer's Attempt: Because the "pop" is random and uncorrelated with the rest of the brain, the Beamformer works its magic. It suppresses the alpha waves, ignores the muscle tension, and puts a red dot exactly on the dysplasia. Victory.

Part 6: The Verdict

We shouldn't view these as "Right vs. Wrong." We should view them as tools on a Synchrony Spectrum.

Use Beamformers when the brain is acting normally, or for very focal, independent spikes. This is the realm of the Asynchronous.

Use LORETA when the brain is seizing, propagating, or acting as a giant connected network. This is the realm of the Hypersynchronous.

The Surgeon's Bottom Line: When I sit down to plan a surgery, I start with LORETA. I need the safety net. I need to see the "blob" to ensure I'm looking at the right lobe. Only then, cautiously, do I switch on the Beamformer—checking constantly to make sure the math hasn't tricked me into seeing a shadow where a fire is burning.

About Author

Azhar ul Haque Sario is a bestselling author and data scientist with a remarkable record of achievement. This Cambridge alumnus brings a wealth of knowledge to his work, holding an MBA (SZABIST), ACCA (Knowledge Level - FTMS College Malaysia and London College of Accountancy, London), BBA, and several Google certifications, including specializations in Google Data Analytics, Google Digital Marketing & E-commerce, and Google Project Management.

With ten years of business experience, Azhar combines practical expertise with his impressive academic background to craft insightful books. His prolific writing has resulted in an astounding 2810 published titles, earning him the record for the maximum Kindle editions and paperback books published by an individual author in one year, awarded by Asia Books of Records in 2024.

ORCID: https://orcid.org/0009-0004-8629-830X
Azhar.sario@hotmail.co.uk
https://www.linkedin.com/in/azharulhaquesario/

www.ingramcontent.com/pod-product-compliance
Lightning Source LLC
Chambersburg PA
CBHW031347230926
51848CB00002B/417
9783384764300